NUDIST CAMP FOLLIES

VOLUME I

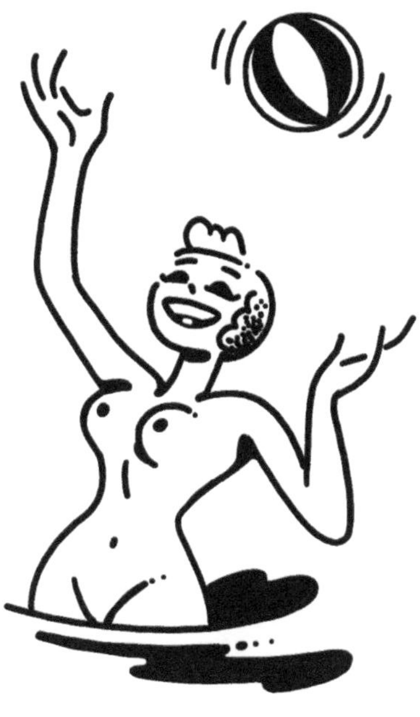

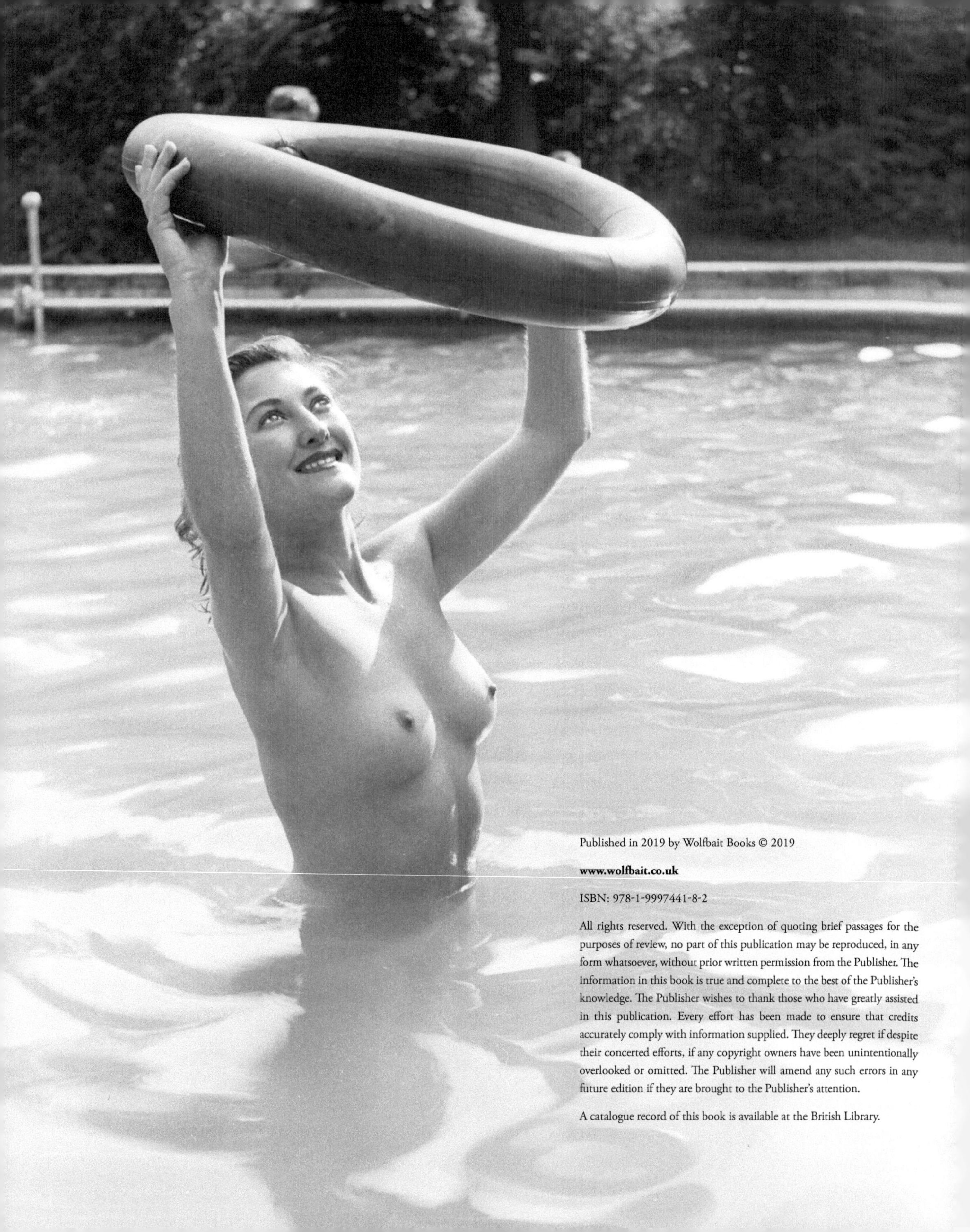

Published in 2019 by Wolfbait Books

www.wolfbait.co.uk

ISBN: 978-1-9997441-8-2

A catalogue record of this book is available at the British Library.

NUDIST CAMP FOLLIES

VOLUME I

By Yahya El-Droubie
Photography by Stephen Glass
Illustrations by Colin Gordon

WOLFBAIT
UNDER THE COUNTER CULTURE

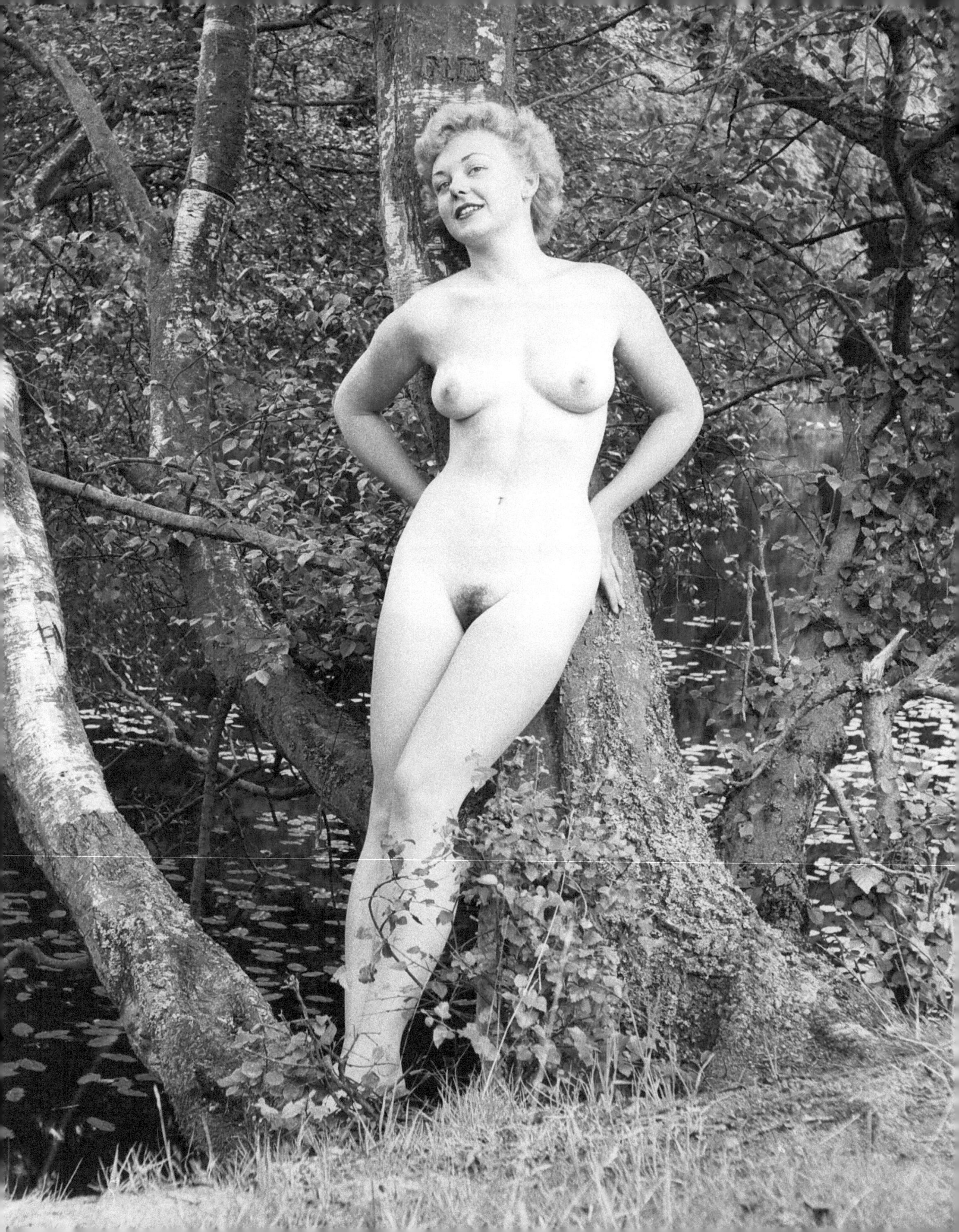

Introduction

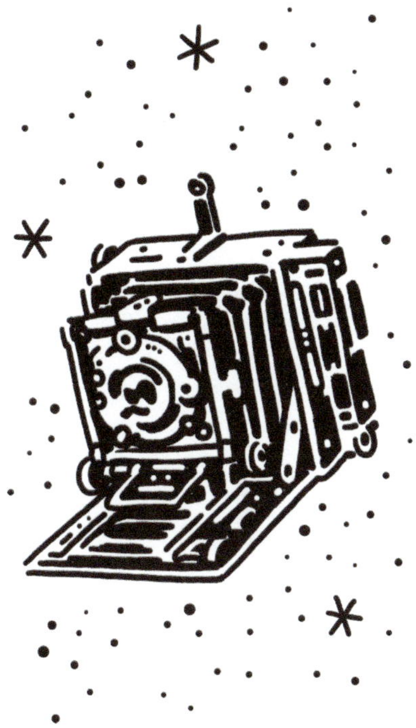

THE PHOTOGRAPHER STEPHEN GLASS is something of an enigma. He was sufficiently well-known during the 1950s for his name to be prominently displayed on magazine covers to help sell them, but very little was written about him or his work at that time. The opposite is true of his elder brother, Zoltán, who was also a photographer. Known to his friends as "Zolly", Zoltán was featured and interviewed in numerous magazines on both sides of the Atlantic.

Zoltán Glass was born in Budapest, Hungary, on April 26, 1903. He began his career as a cartoonist and retoucher for a local newspaper, but in 1925 he moved to Berlin, where he was employed as the picture editor of an evening newspaper; he then moved on to the *Berliner Tagblatt* as a photojournalist. Zoltán prospered and was soon able to develop a thriving freelance business as a commercial photographer and journalist. He established Reclaphot, a photographic agency that specialised in advertising work, and Autophot, a company dedicated exclusively to automobile photography. A keen motor sport enthusiast and amateur racer, Zoltán covered Germany's biggest races at the Nürburgring and Avus circuits. His famous photographs are of the Mercedes-Benz Silver Arrows team, which dominated Grand Prix racing in the mid-1930s.

With the rise of Hitler, business became increasingly difficult in Germany, and Zoltán fled to London. As an enemy alien at the outbreak of World War II, he was not permitted to pursue his profession and faced the threat of internment, so he voluntarily handed over his camera equipment to the British authorities.

After the war, Zoltán eked out a living taking publicity stills for clients in the film and theatre worlds. His career took a big step up when fellow Hungarian Arpad Elfer, Creative Director of Colman, Prentis & Varley, one of the most prestigious London ad agencies, started giving him work. By the mid-1950s, he was one of the most successful fashion and advertising photographers in the capital, with a studio at 183 Kings Road, Chelsea, and later another at 41 Paradise Walk, SW3.

Nudism is not a religious movement; it embraces members of all denominations including clergymen of the Church of England and nonconformist ministers.

— William Welby, The Naked Truth about Nudism, 1941.

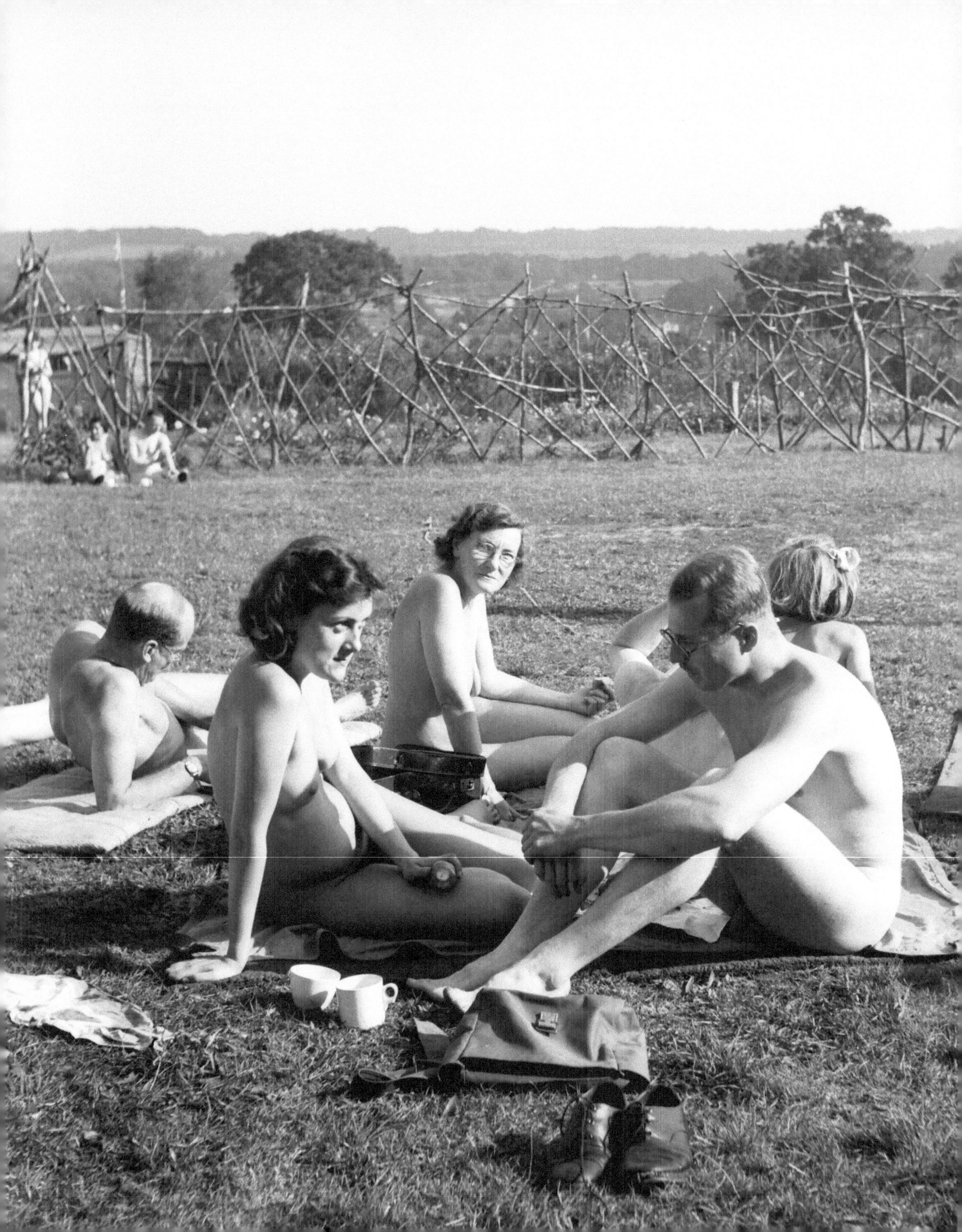

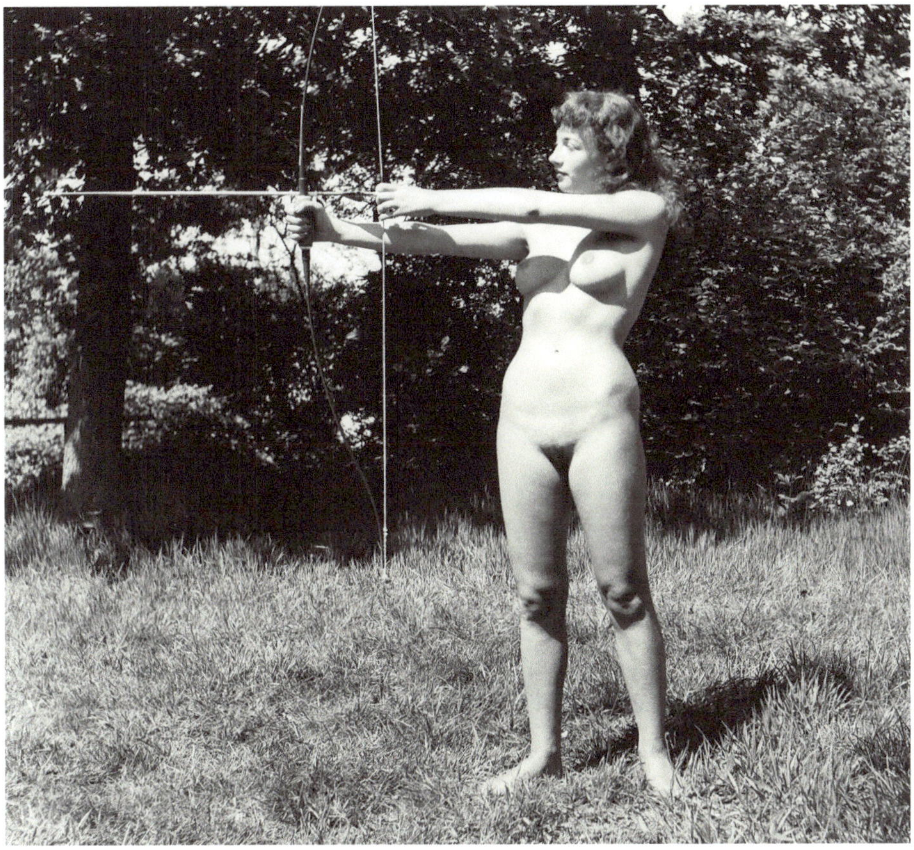

After the war, we saw a new type of person becoming interested in nudism. Previously it had always been the well-to-do, educated, rather out-of-the-ordinary type of person who joined the movement. Now we began to see the average, unprejudiced Englishman and his wife.
– Dorothy Macaskie

Left: Model Pamela Green poses as Artemis, the Greek goddess of the hunt, at Spielplatz nudist camp in 1951.

One of his clients was Odhams Press, who published *Lilliput*, a pocket-sized gentleman's magazine that featured an assortment of titillating articles and risqué humour, together with adventurous photographic essays from such well-known talents as Bill Brandt and Brassai.

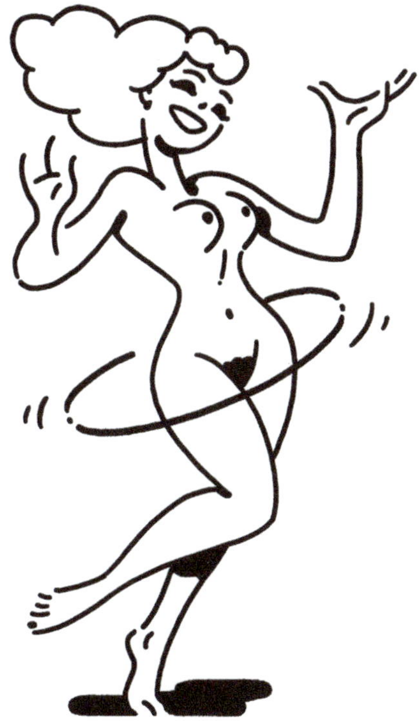

Zoltán's brother, Stephen, who also fled Europe during World War II, carved out a name for himself taking pictures for such publications as *The Naturist* and *Health and Efficiency.* The well-known model Pamela Green (1929–2010) posed for him several times at the infamous nudist camp Spielplatz in Bricket Wood, Hertfordshire, and at his tiny first-floor studio in Old Church Street, just off the Kings Road in Chelsea. *"In those days, when Stephen photographed me, I still had dark hair. He liked his props, especially stuffed animals,"* she said. Pamela's agent, Pearl Beresford, sent her along to Zoltán, whose studio on the Kings Road was enormous by comparison. Unlike Stephen, Zoltán was brisk and businesslike.

Iseult, the daughter of Spielplatz co-founders Charles and Dorothy Macaskie, remembers Stephen. *"He would often ask me to pose for him,"* she said. *"I quite*

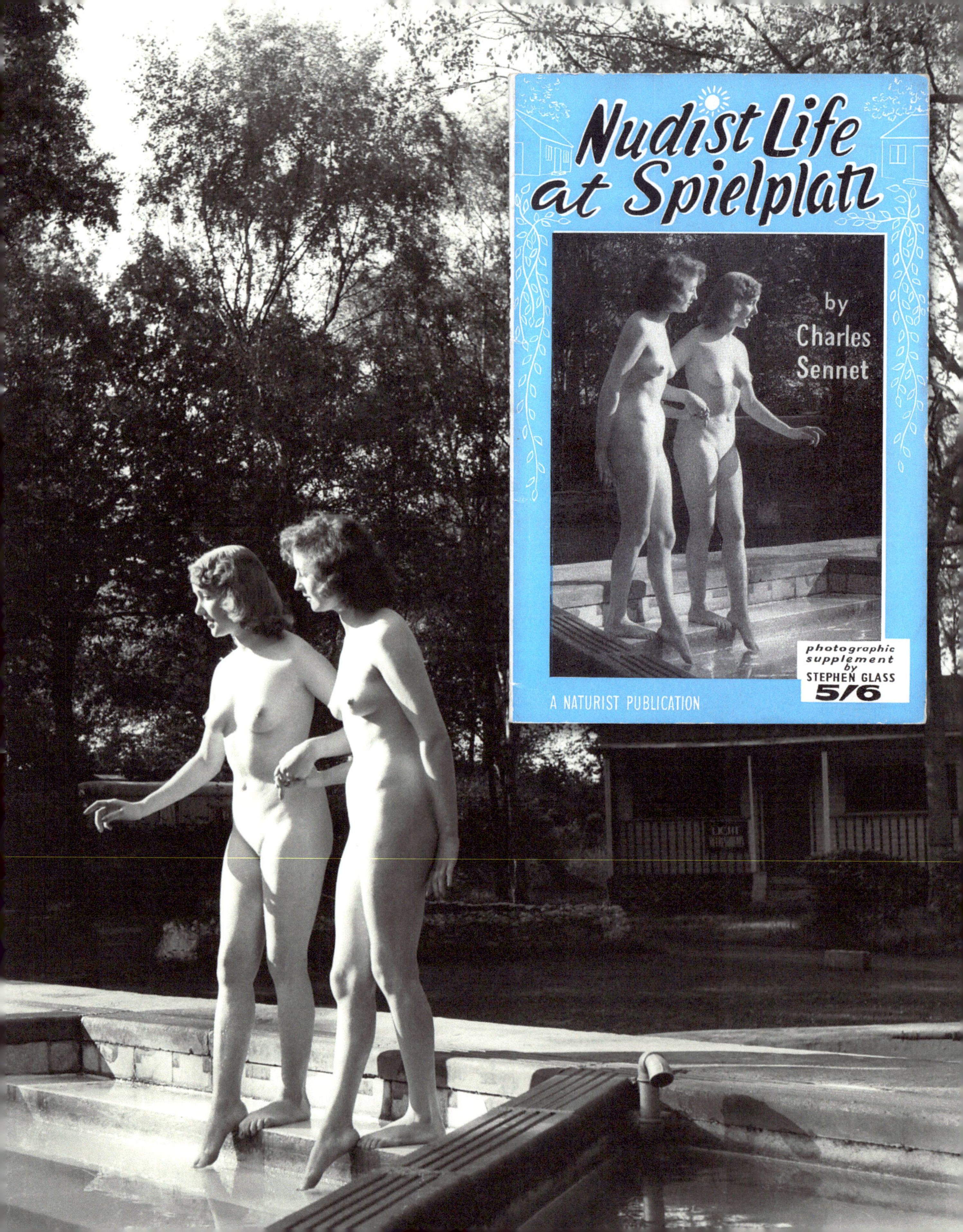
Nudist Life
at Spielplatz
by
Charles
Sennet
photographic
supplement
by
STEPHEN GLASS
5/6
A NATURIST PUBLICATION

enjoyed having my photo taken, but when I asked to be paid, he stopped using me. A bit of pocket money back then would have been nice."

As well as magazines, Stephen's work graced a series of small books published by The Naturist Ltd., such as *Sussex Maidens* (1949), *The Pool of Enchantment* (1950) and *Nudist Life in Spielplatz* (1956). He also photographed the popular model June Palmer (1940–2004). The photos in this book are from his uncensored negatives.

Until the end of the 1960s, it was considered obscene to show pubic hair or genitalia in British publications. To ensure an image of a naked young lady would not incur the wrath of the censor, the model would shave down below and the photograph would then be retouched by hand to erase anything problematic.

By 1964, Zoltán Glass had made enough money to sell his Chelsea studios to a consortium of British photographers. He then moved to a villa in Roquebrune on the French Riviera, with his common-law wife Pat, a former cabaret dancer. He offered his collection of pin-up photography to glamour photographer Harrison Marks who, strangely, turned it down. Zoltán died in France on February 24, 1981, at the age of 78, leaving neither offspring nor a will. His photographs were eventually given to The National Science and Media Museum in Bradford, Yorkshire. Stephen Glass died on 23 April, 1990. His work ended up at auction.

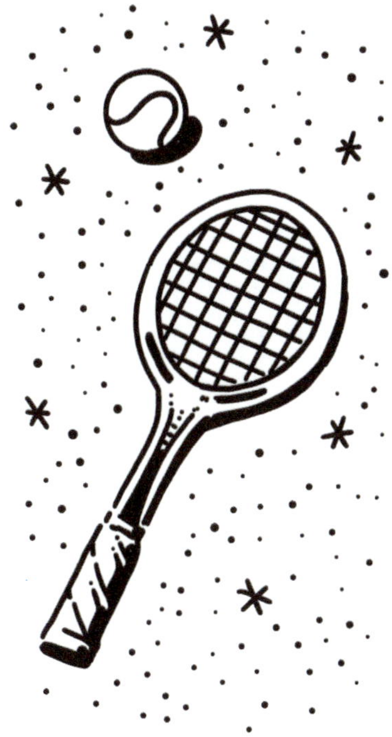

Just outside London, between Watford and St Albans, there are four nudist camps: Fiveacres Country Club, established in 1927; Spielplatz, established in 1929; Sun Folk Society, established in 1931 and Diogenes, founded in 1932. All the camps have proved popular with photographers over the years, especially Spielplatz, which is a naturist village with permanent residents.

Spielplatz was founded by Charles Macaskie and his wife Dorothy, who moved from London to an area of virgin woodland they purchased near the village of Bricket Wood in Hertfordshire. Their daughter, Iseult, and granddaughter still live there today. Among Spielplatz's notable members was Ross Nichols, founder of the Order of Bards, Ovates and Druids; he in turn attracted Gerald Gardner, who in his development of Wicca, established his first coven at Bricket Wood.

Left: *Nudist Life at Spielplatz* – Charles Sennet's book telling the story of a modern experiment in the art of living – alongside the original negative of the cover image. As you can see, the publisher flipped the image for the cover. The book came with an art supplement of photographs taken at the Hertfordshire nudist resort by Stephen Glass. It was published by The Naturist Ltd. in 1956.

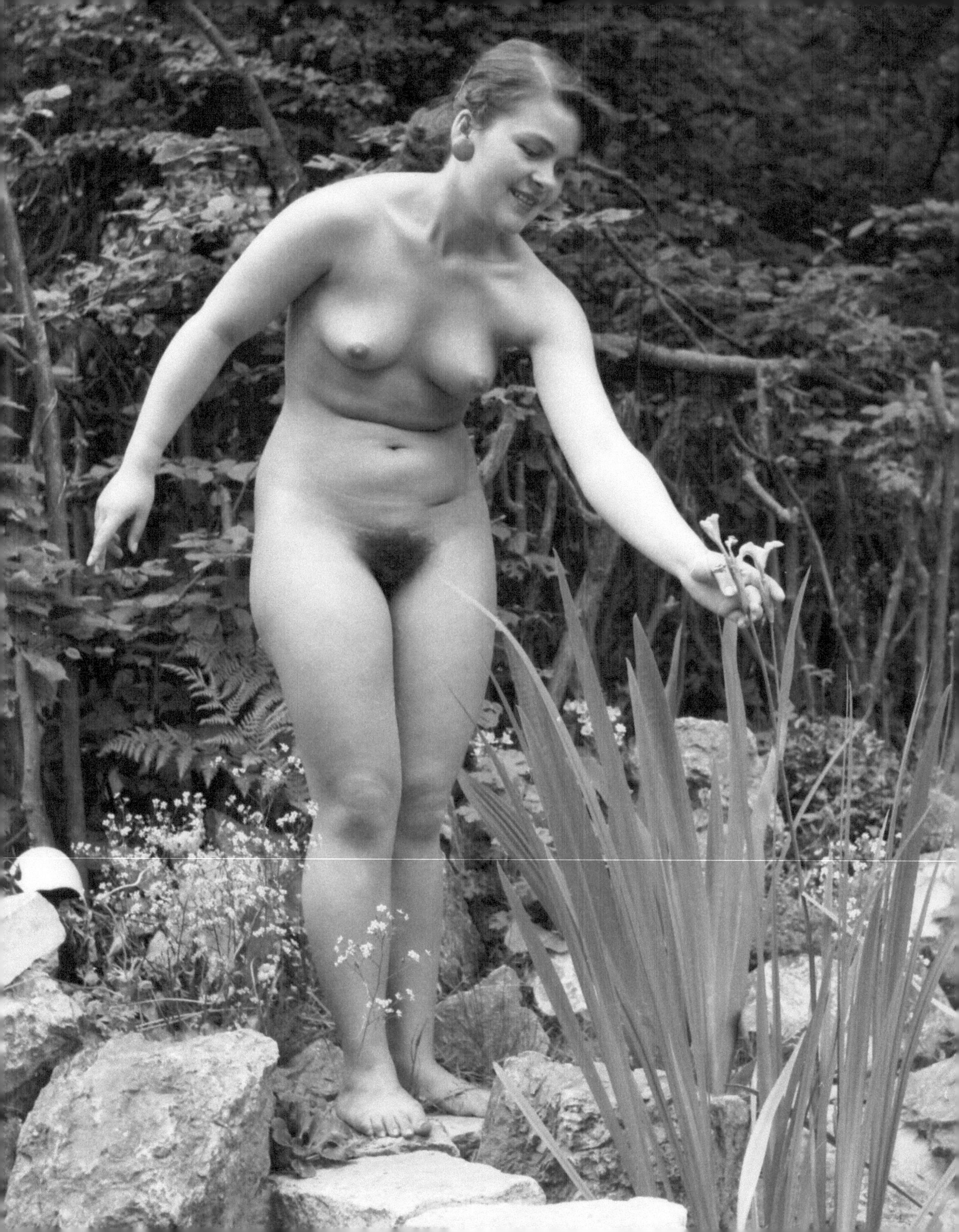

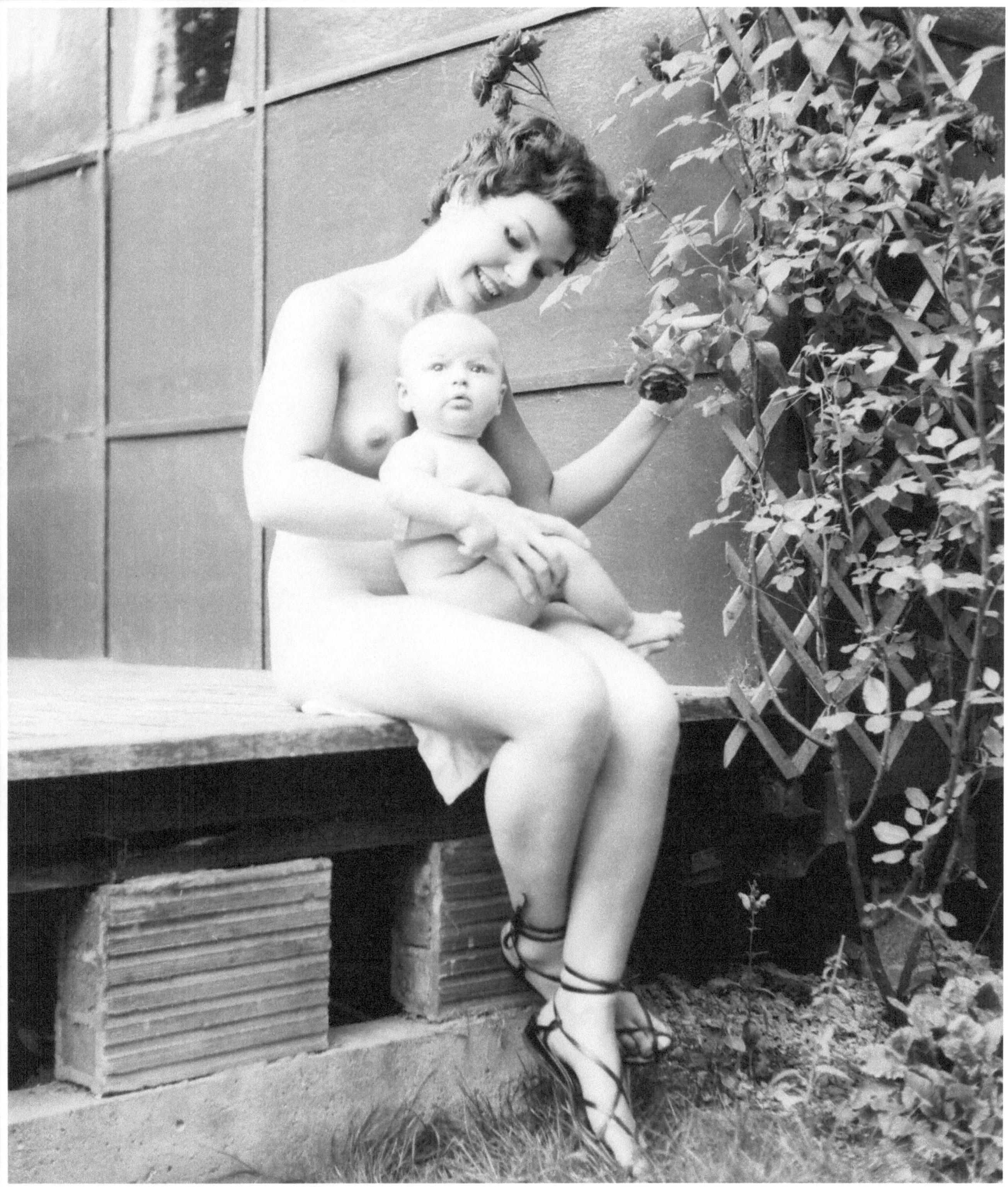

Left: Zettie, Iseult's younger sister.
Above: Iseult and her daughter Beverly in 1955.

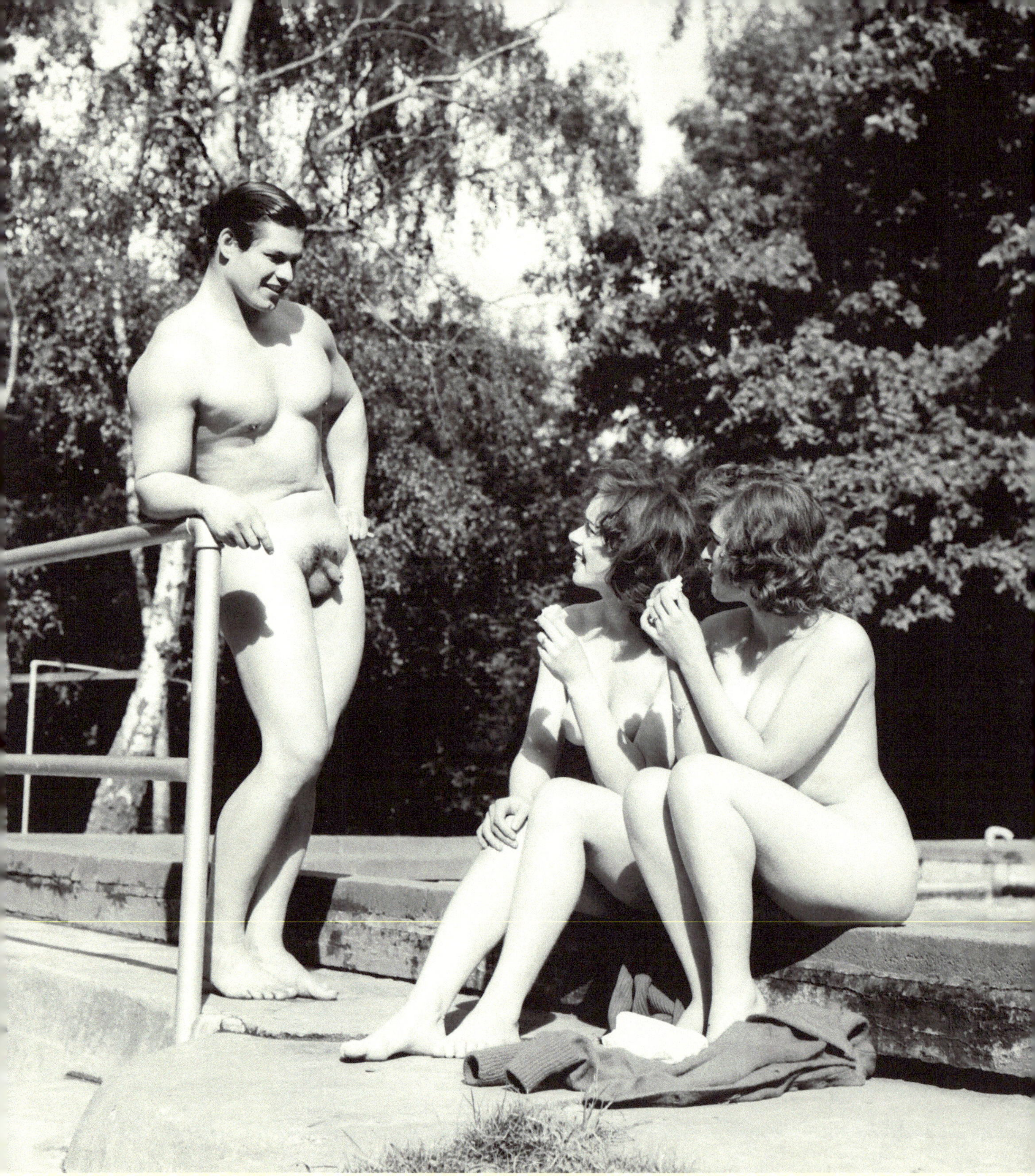

Right: Audrey Wayne and Anita Smith.

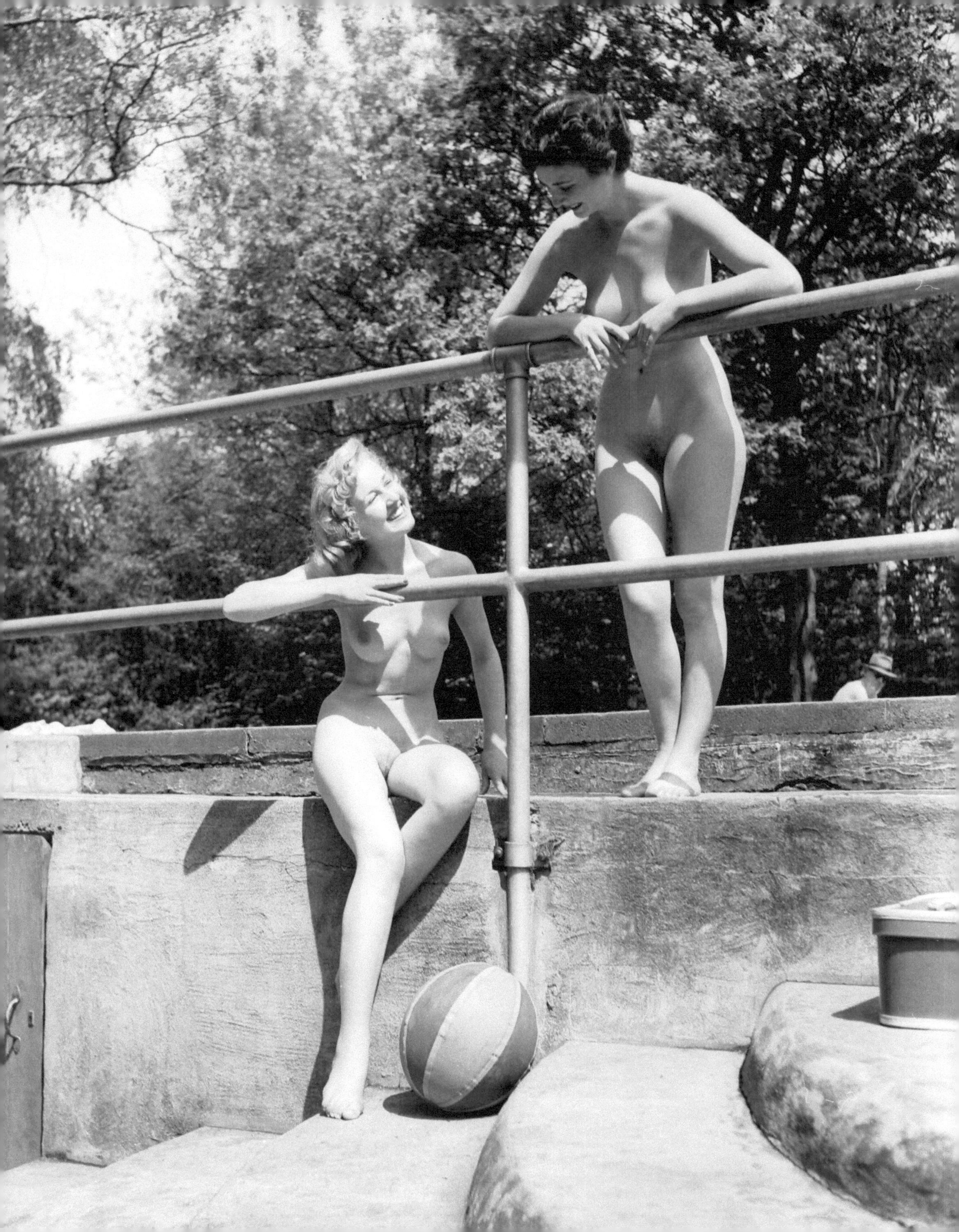

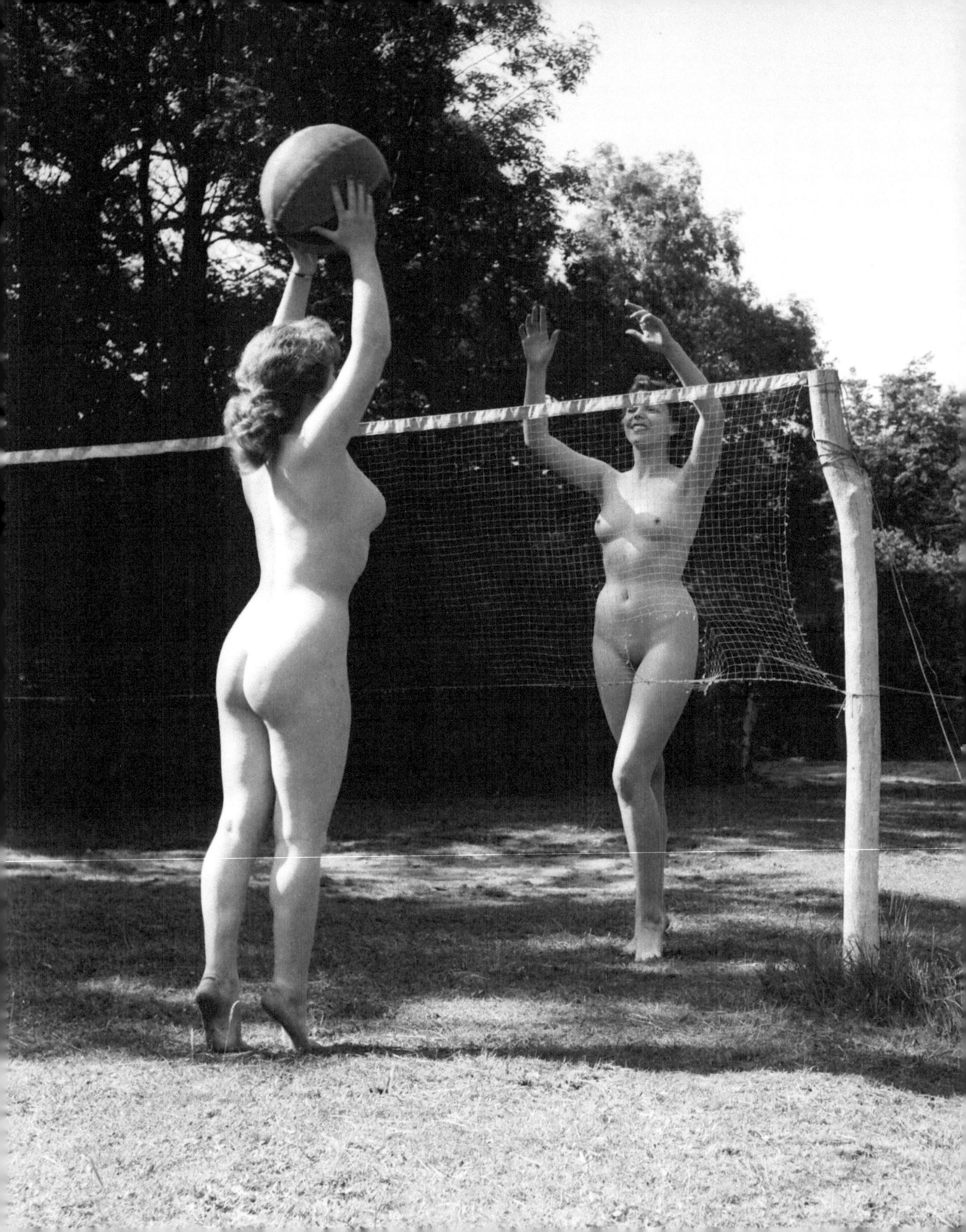

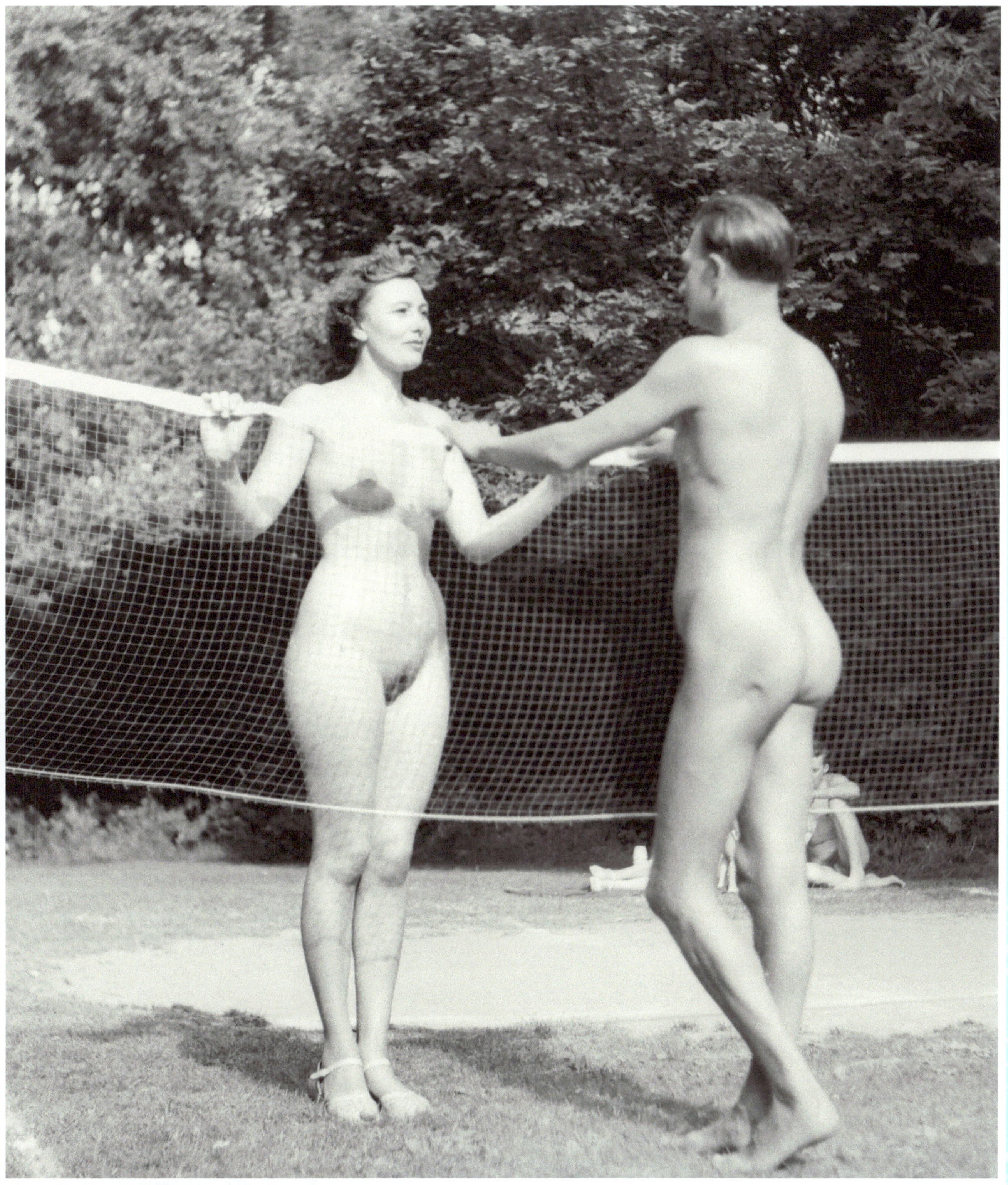

Left and above: These images from *Nudist Life at Spielplatz* were captioned: "Ever played volleyball in clothes? Then you will appreciate at once the advantages of *this* mode of play."

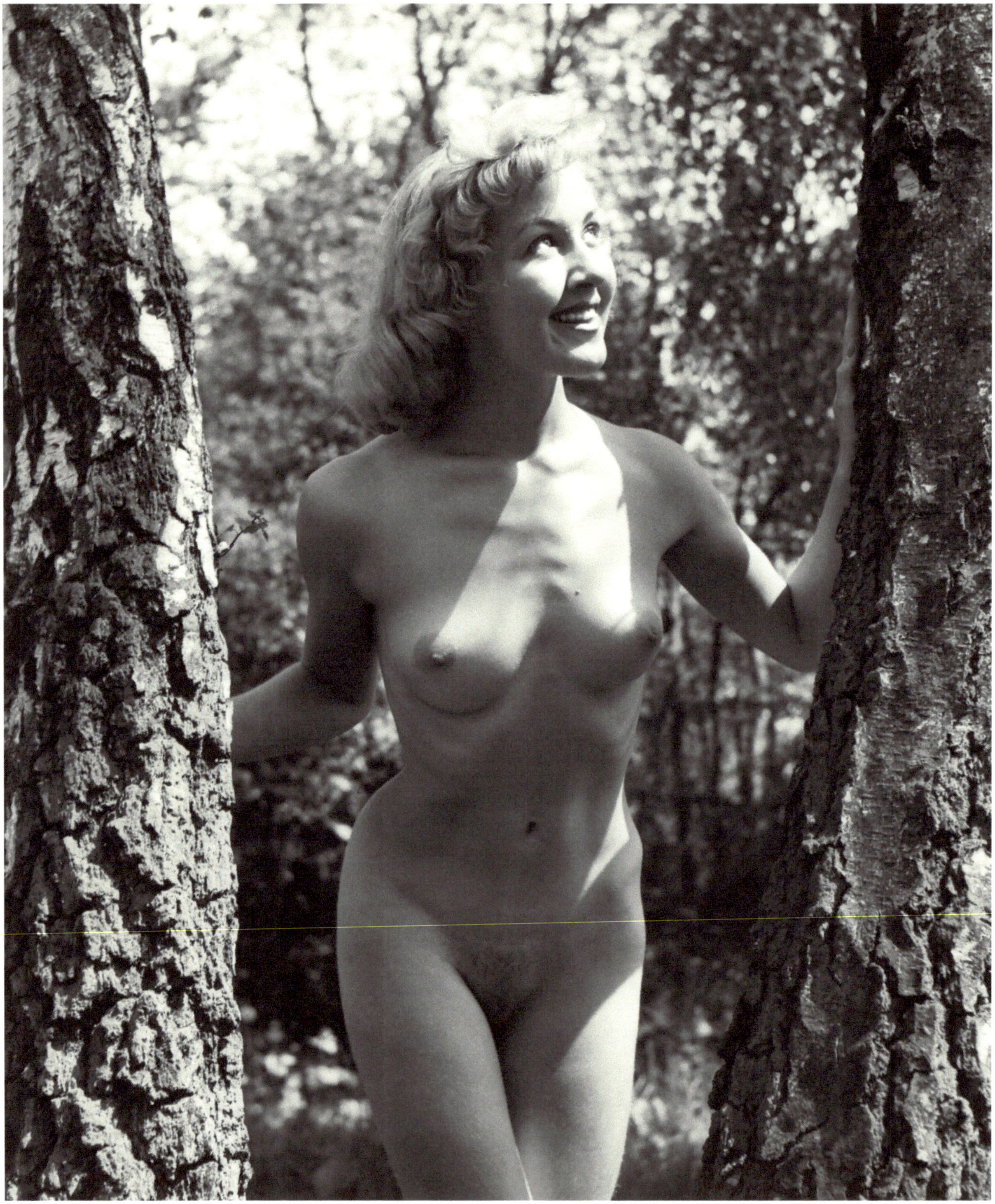

Above and right: Audrey Wayne.

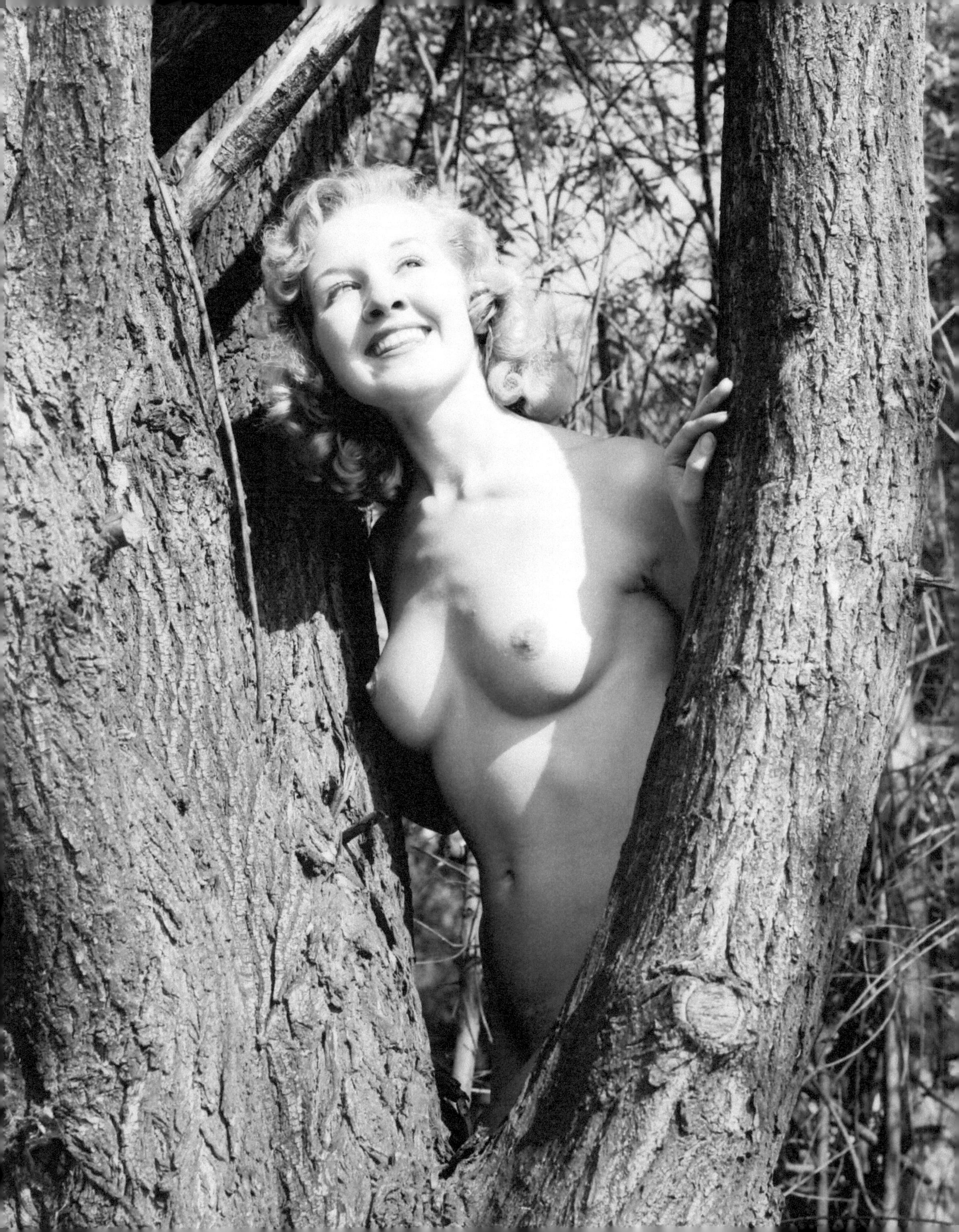

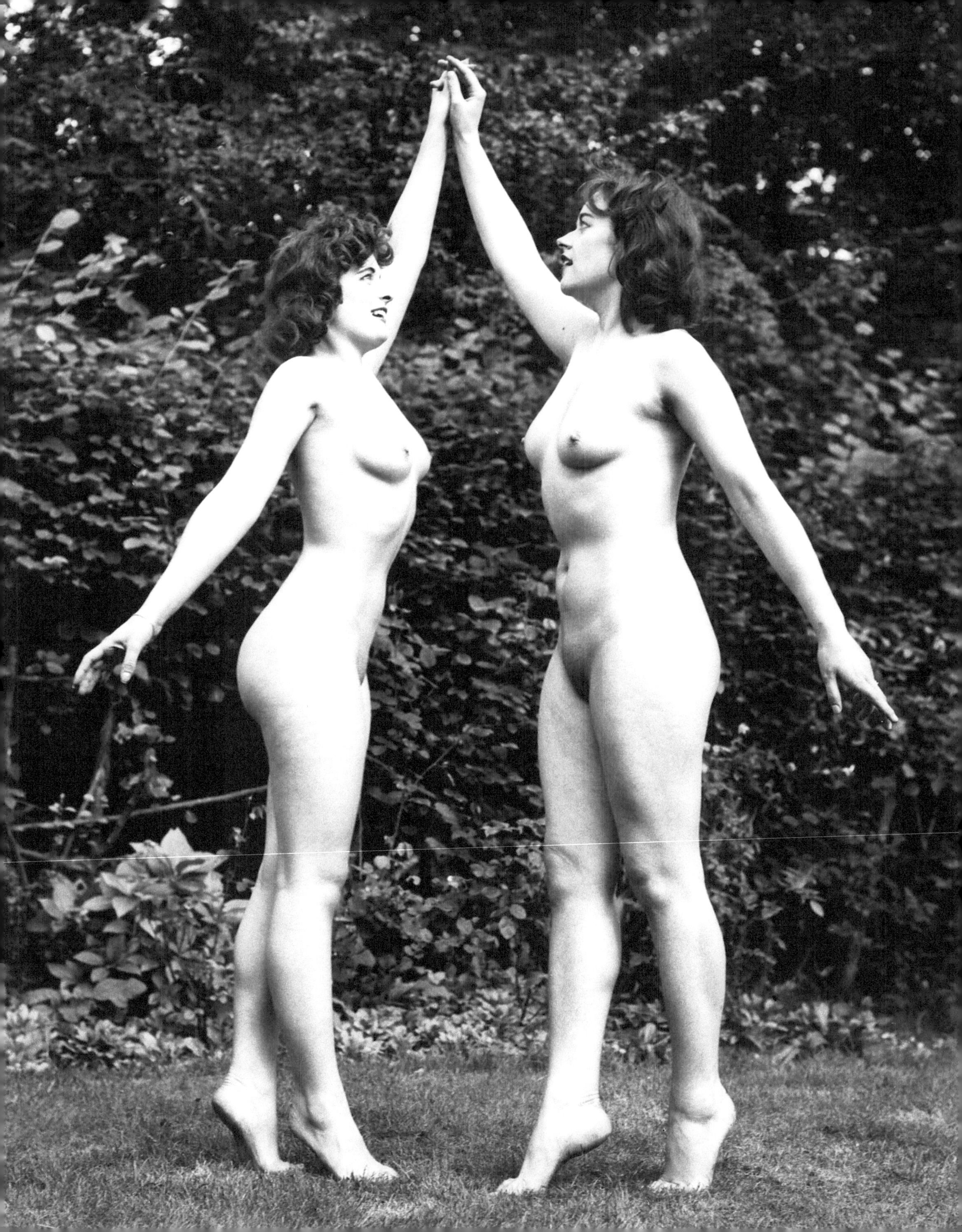

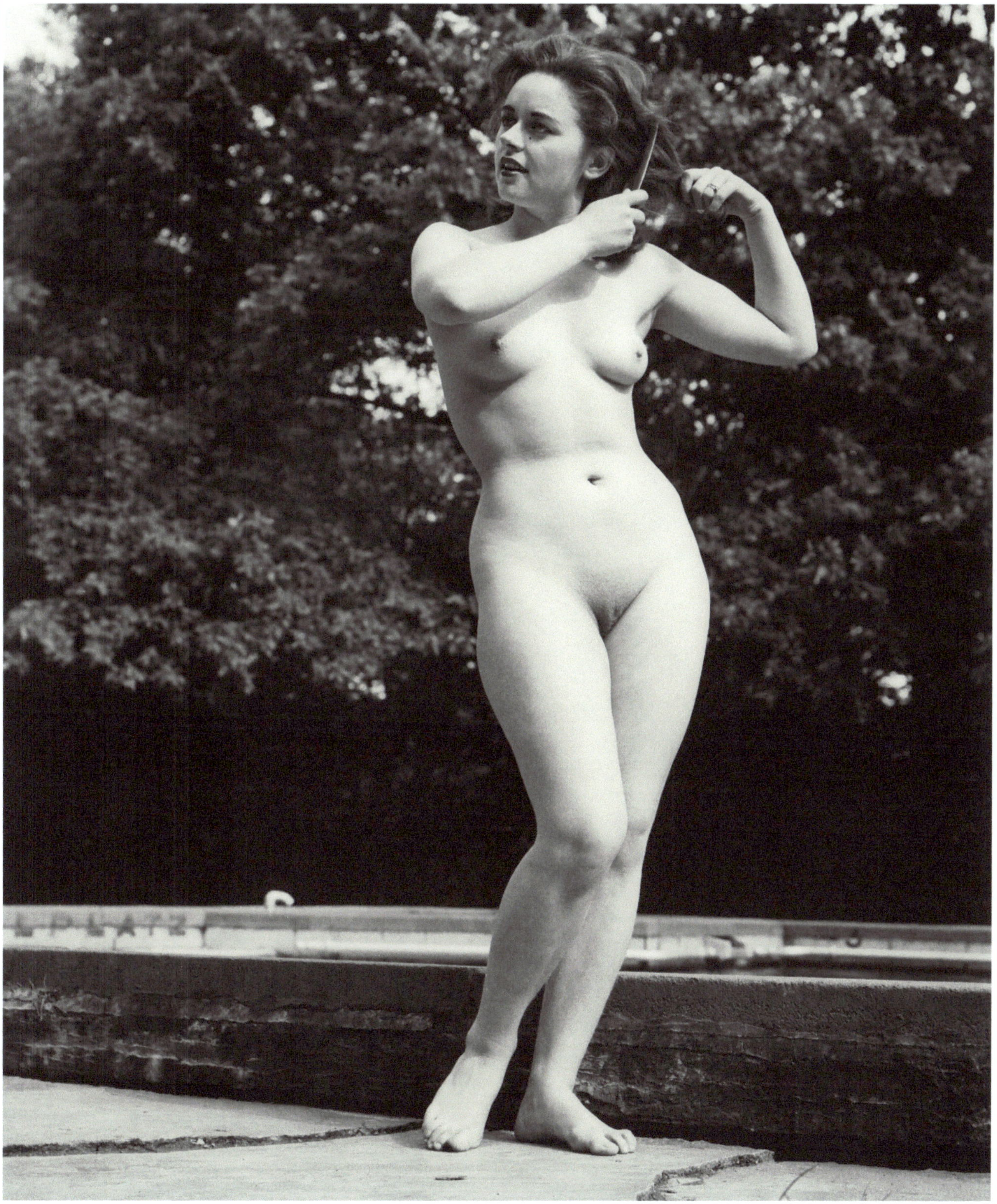

Above: Mary Corbet.

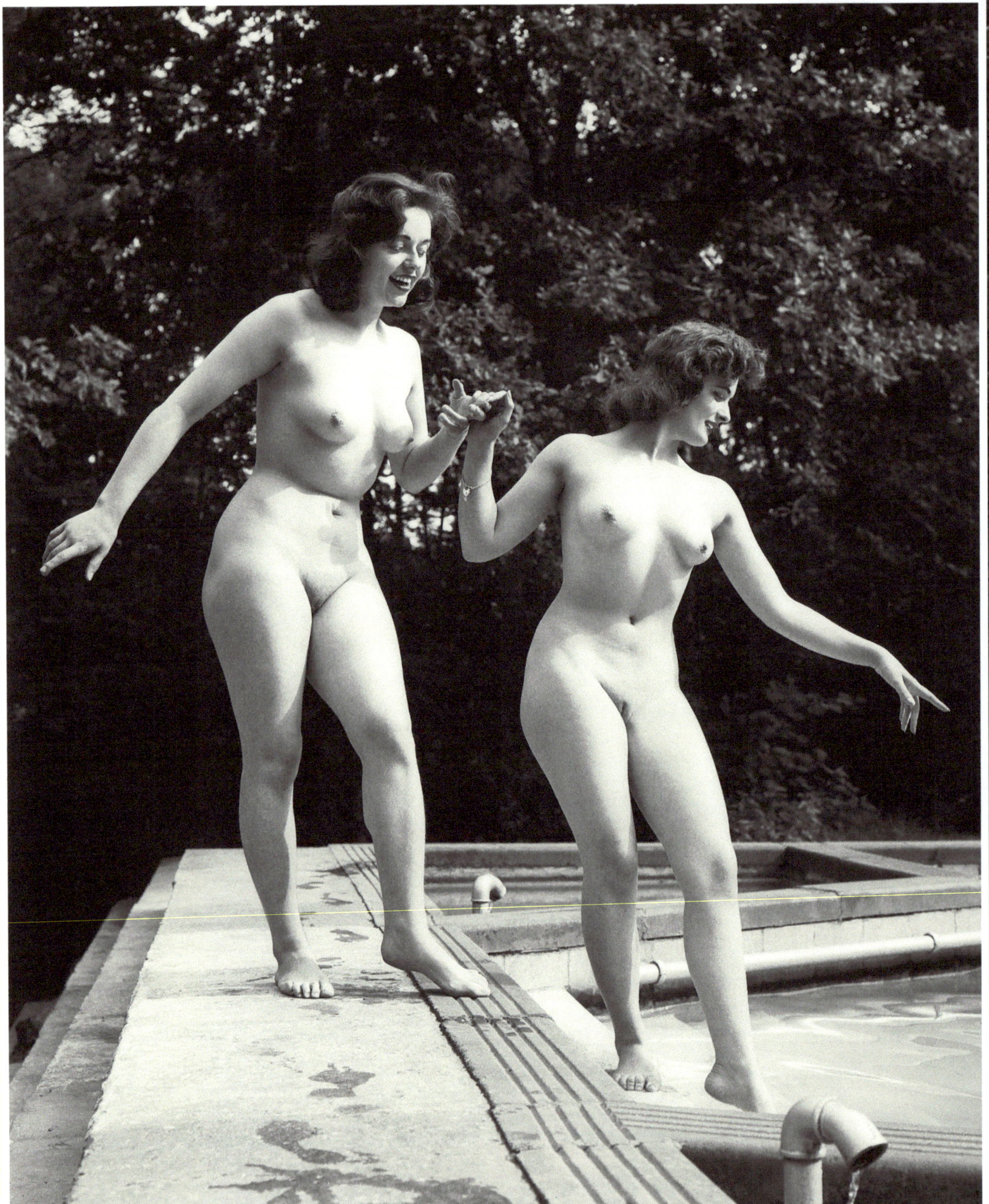

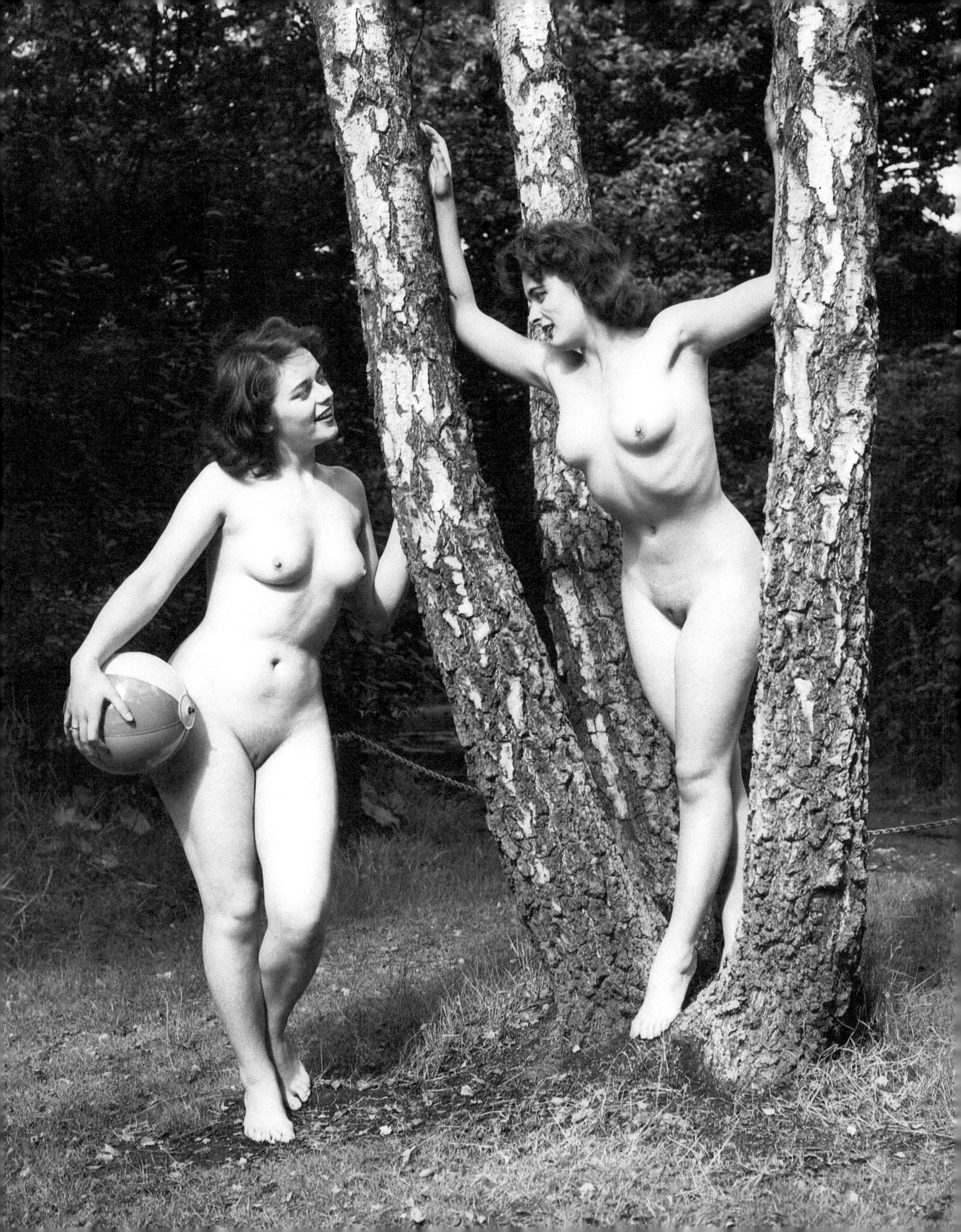

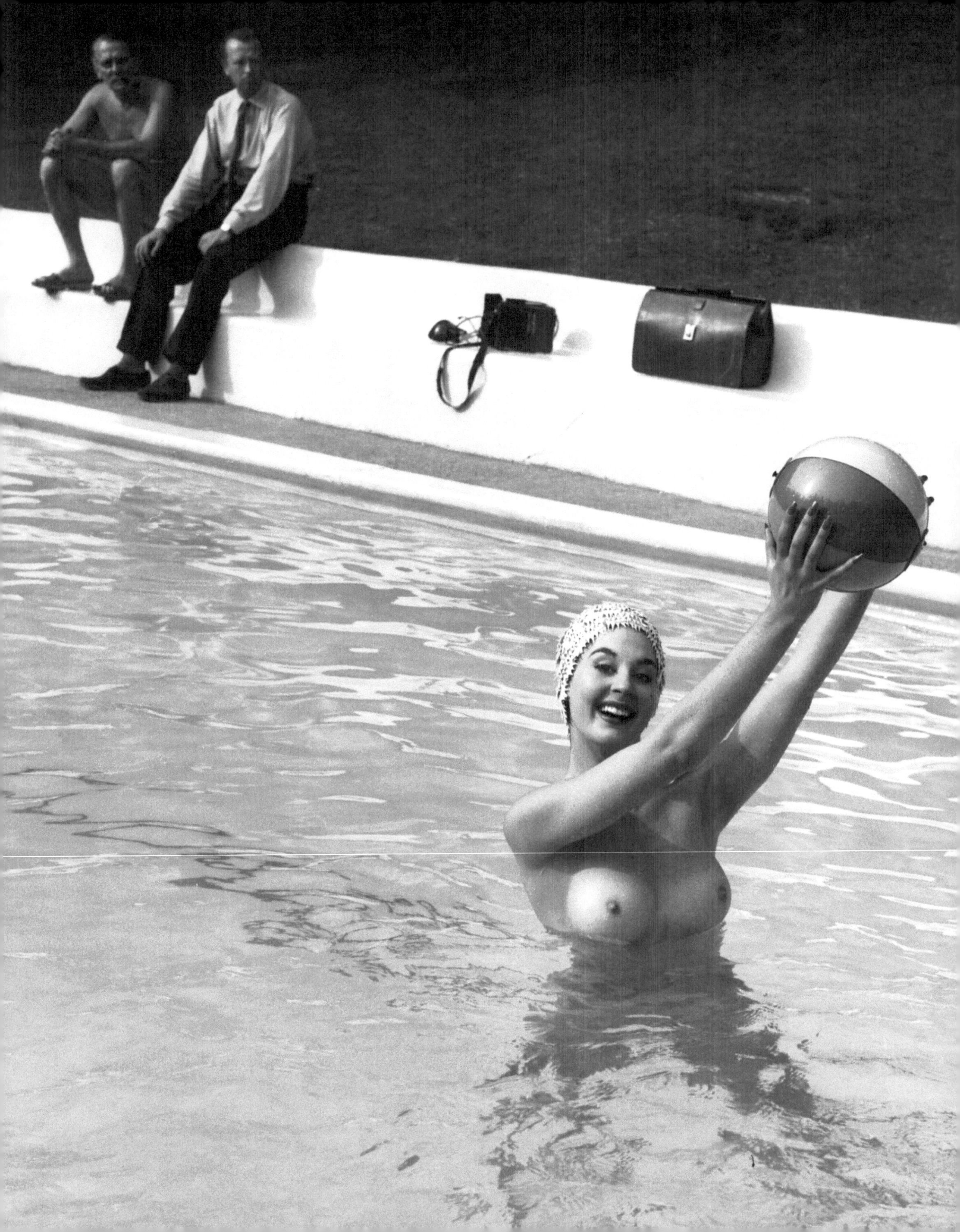

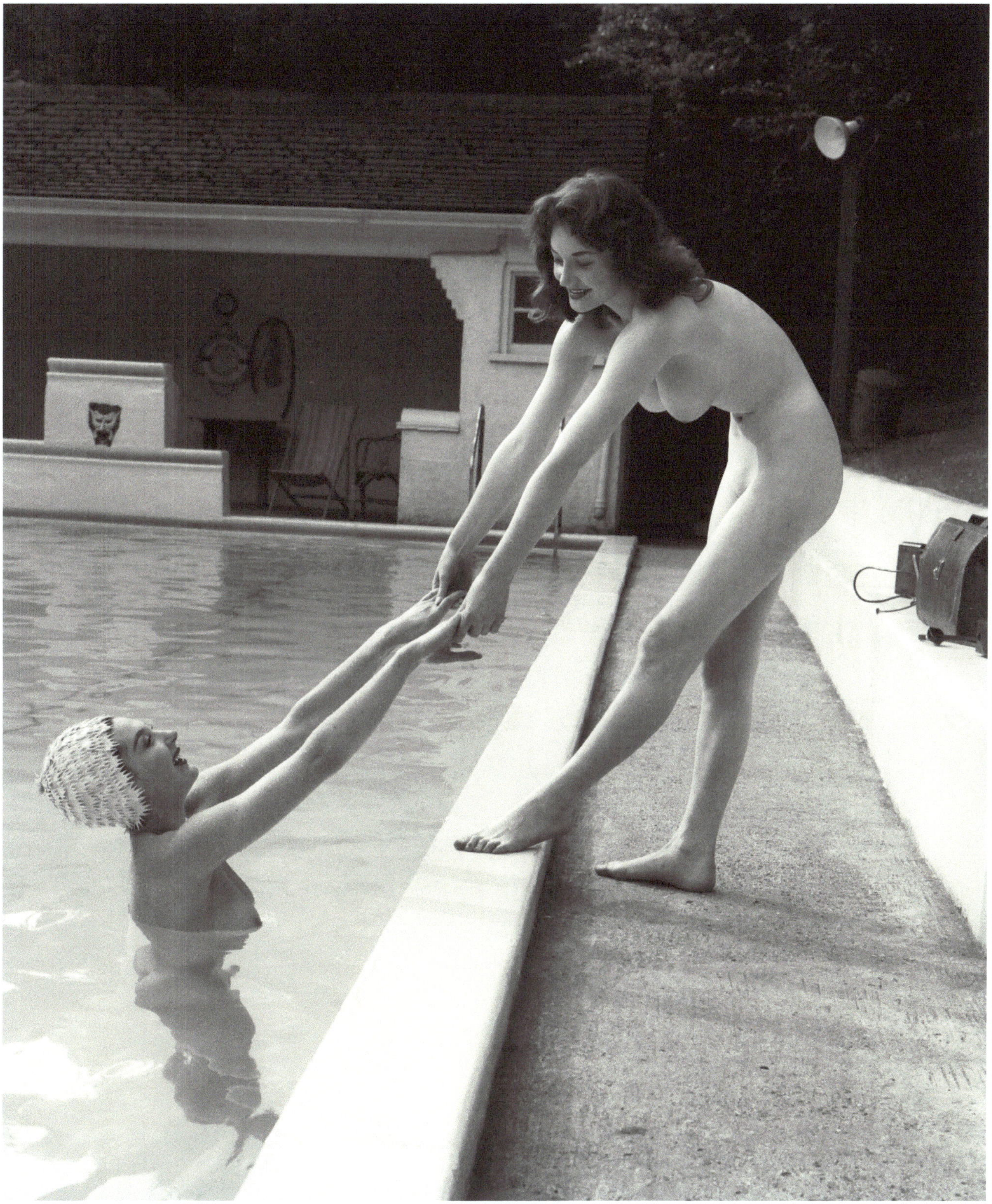

Left and Above: The outdoor pool at the White House, a tranquil naturist haven, set in a wooded valley near Caterham, Surrey, that was founded in 1933.

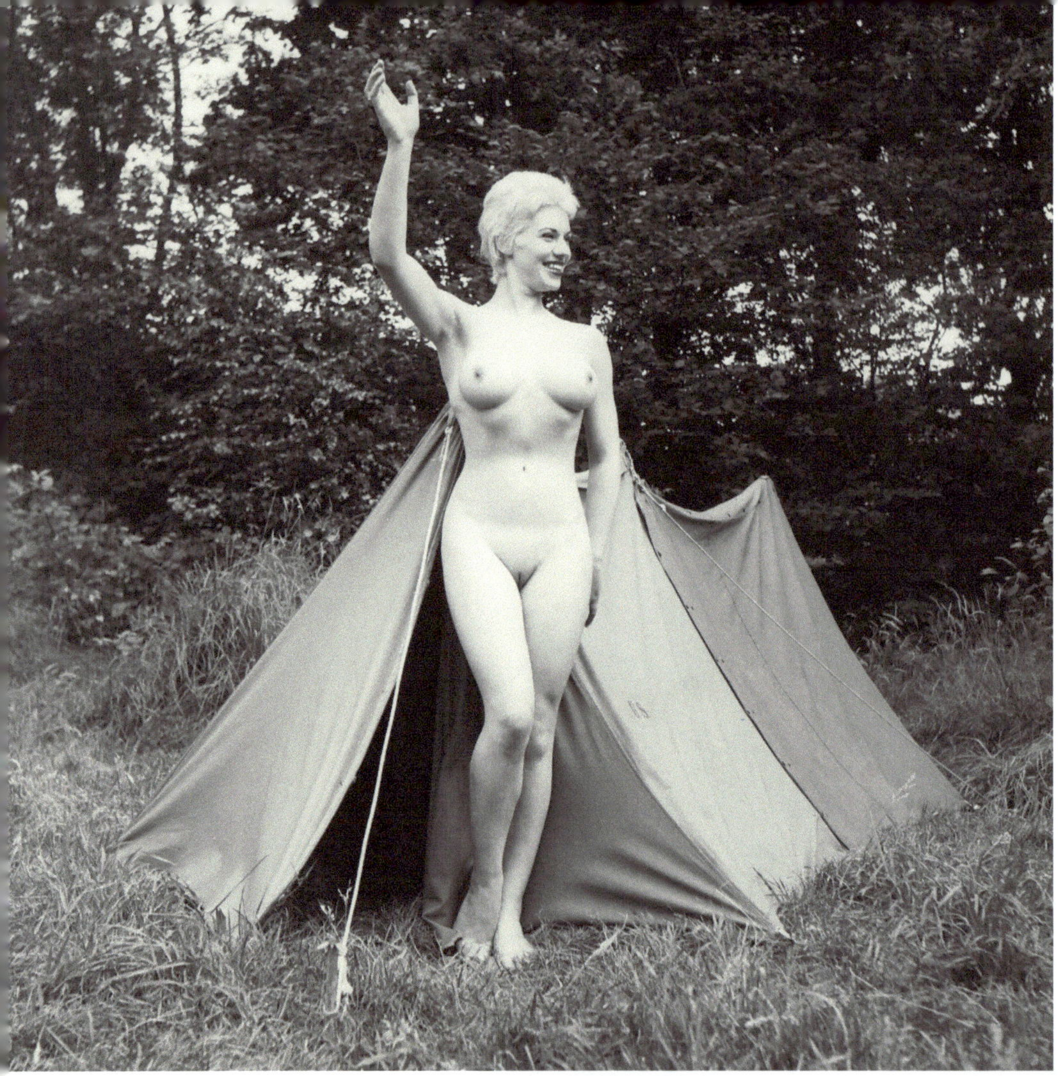

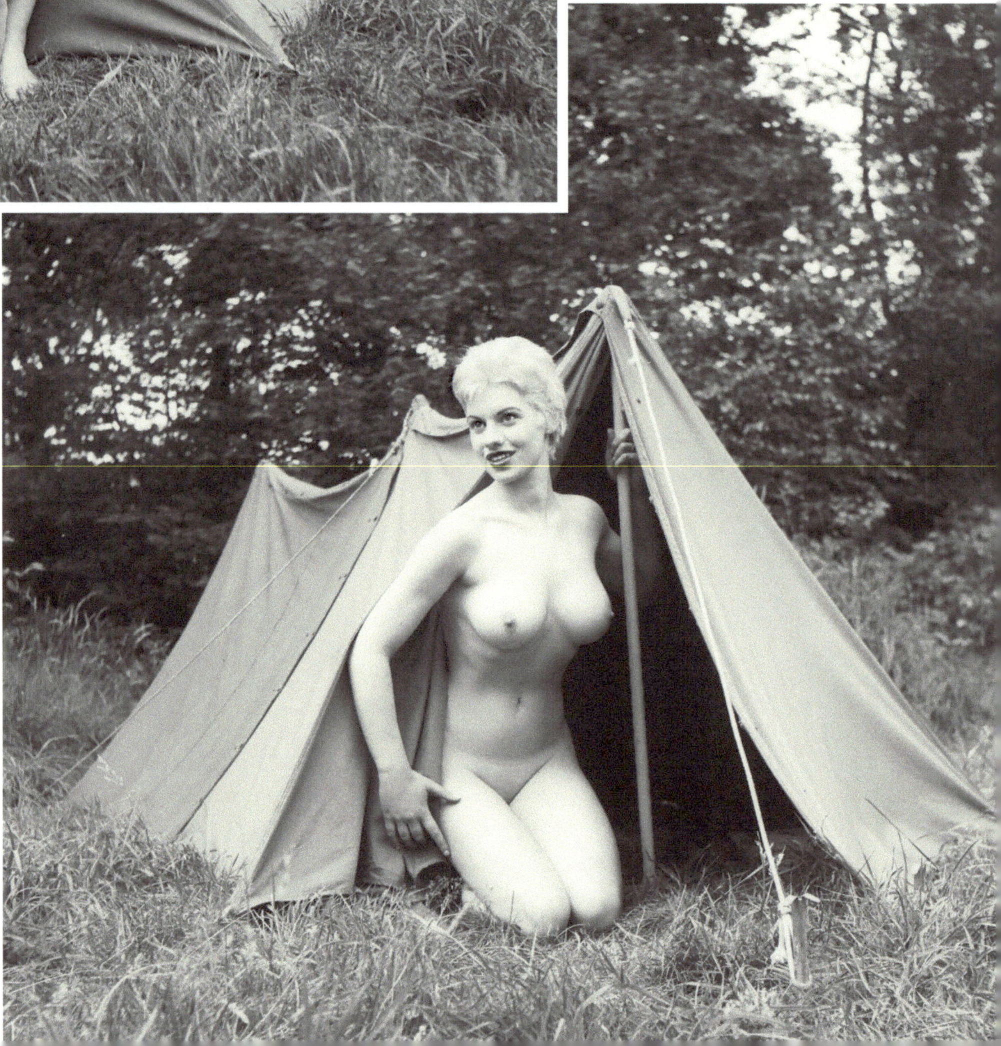

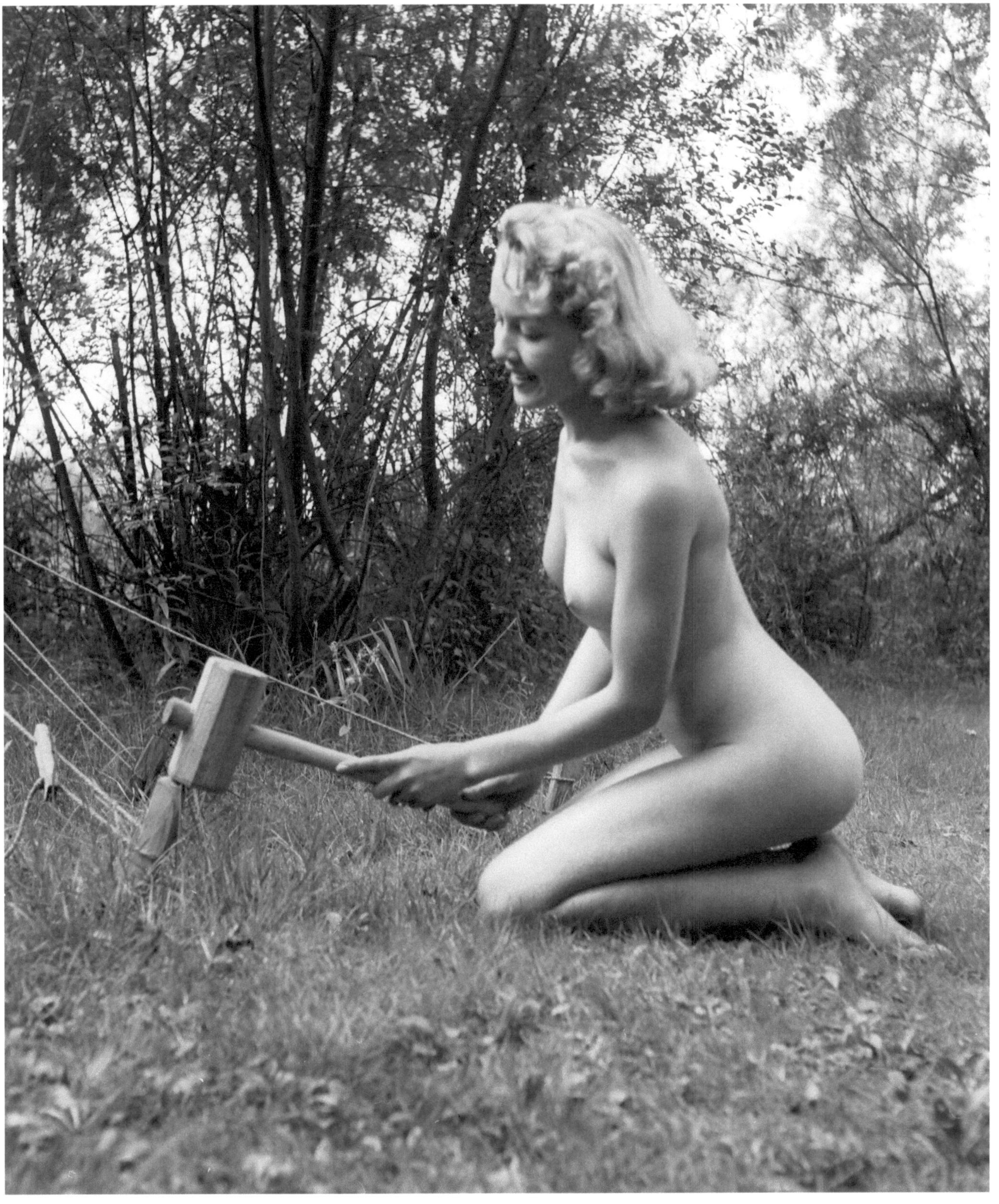

Left: Kim Foster. **Above:** Audrey Wayne.

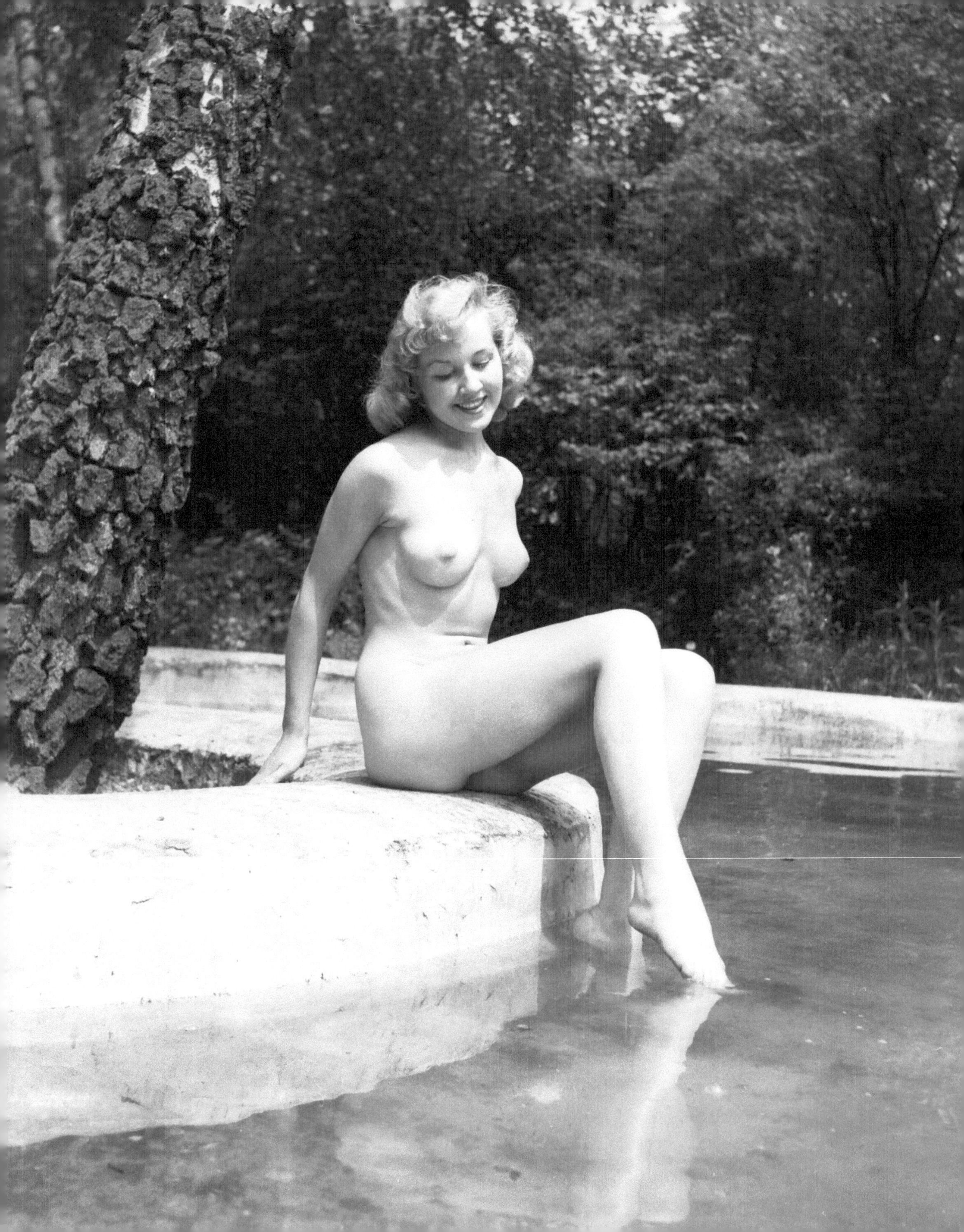

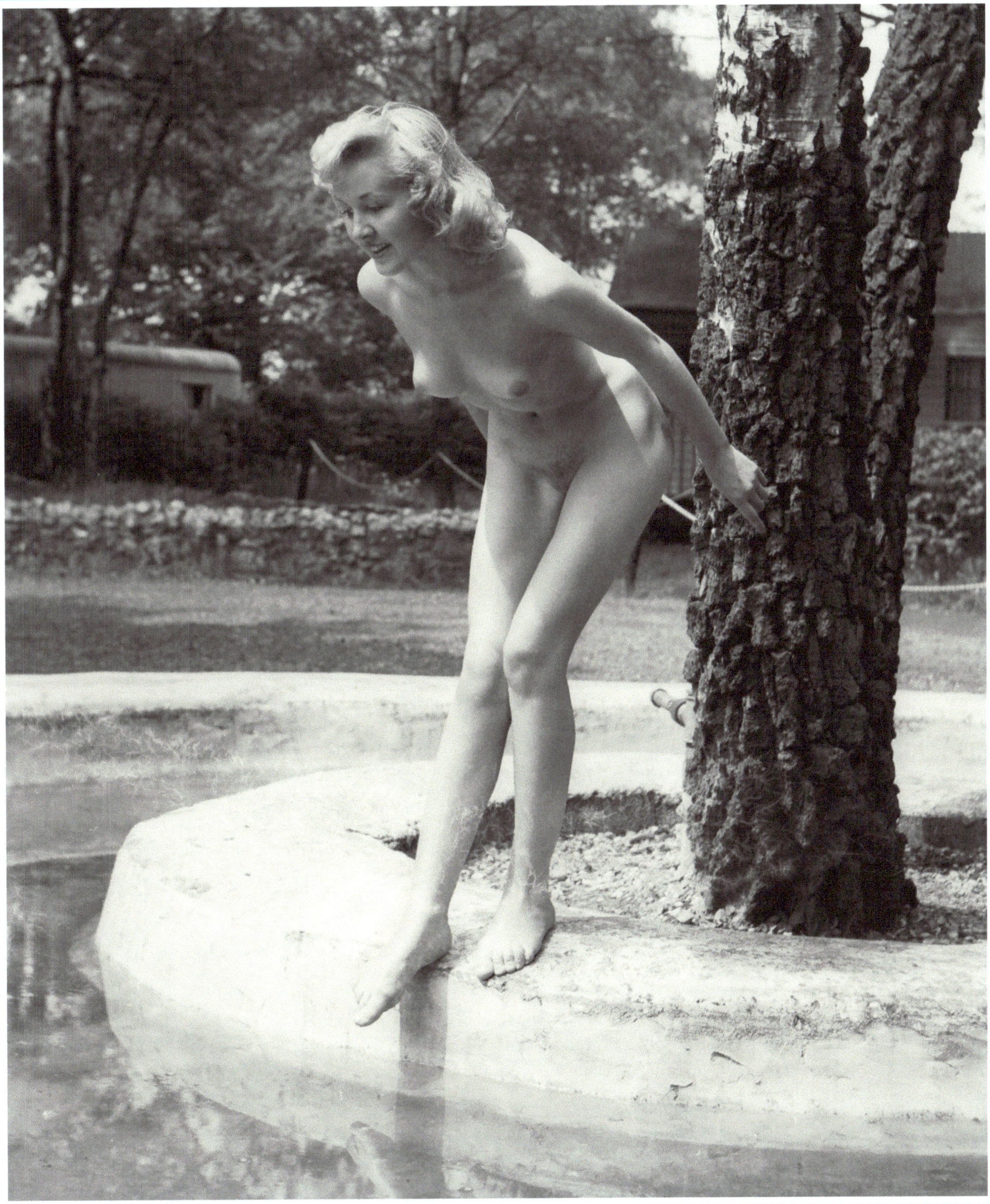

Left: Audrey Wayne. **Above:** This shot of Audrey Wayne appeared on the cover of *The Mystery of Naturism* by Melvyn Oakdale, The Naturist Ltd., 1956.

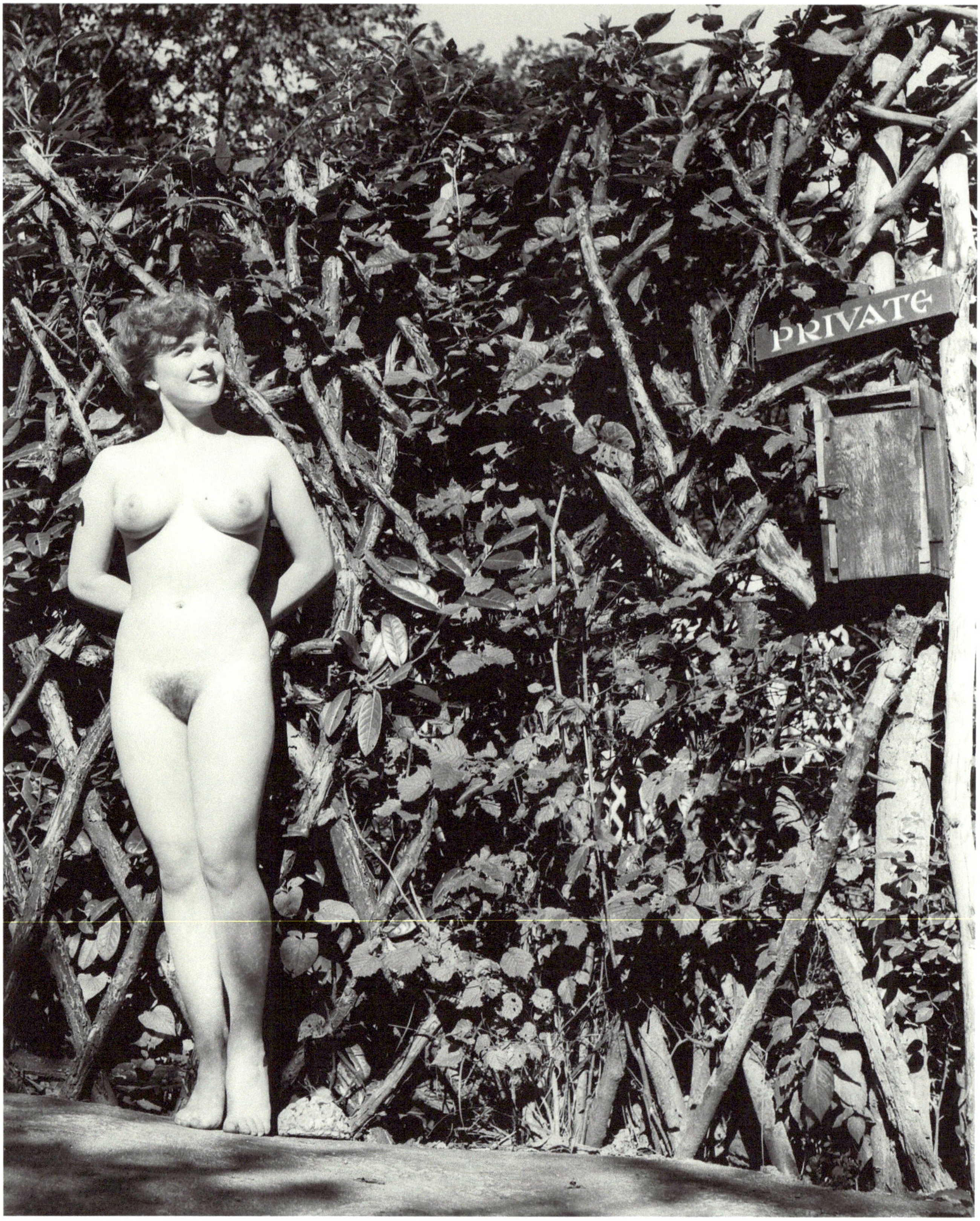
PRIVATE

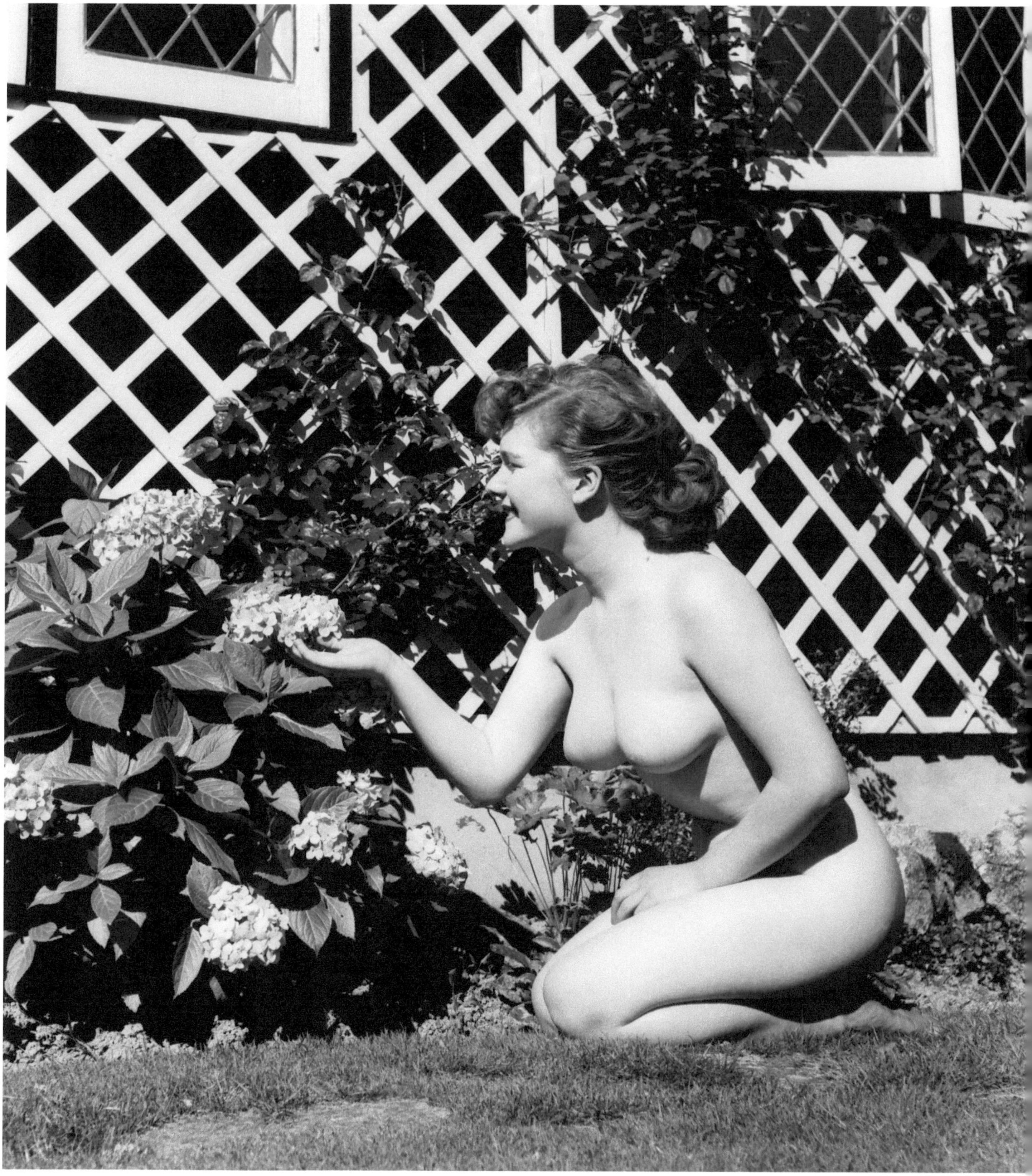

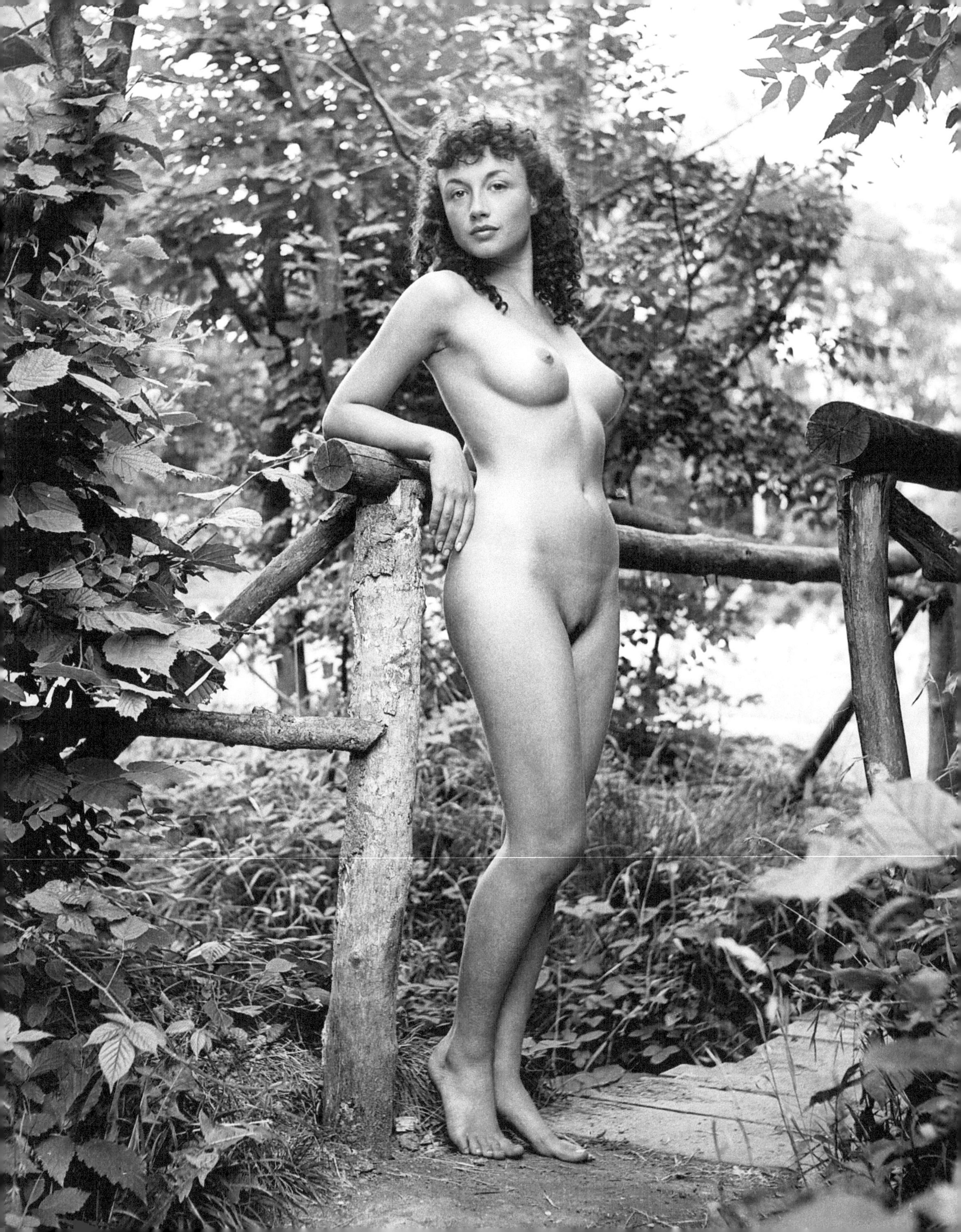

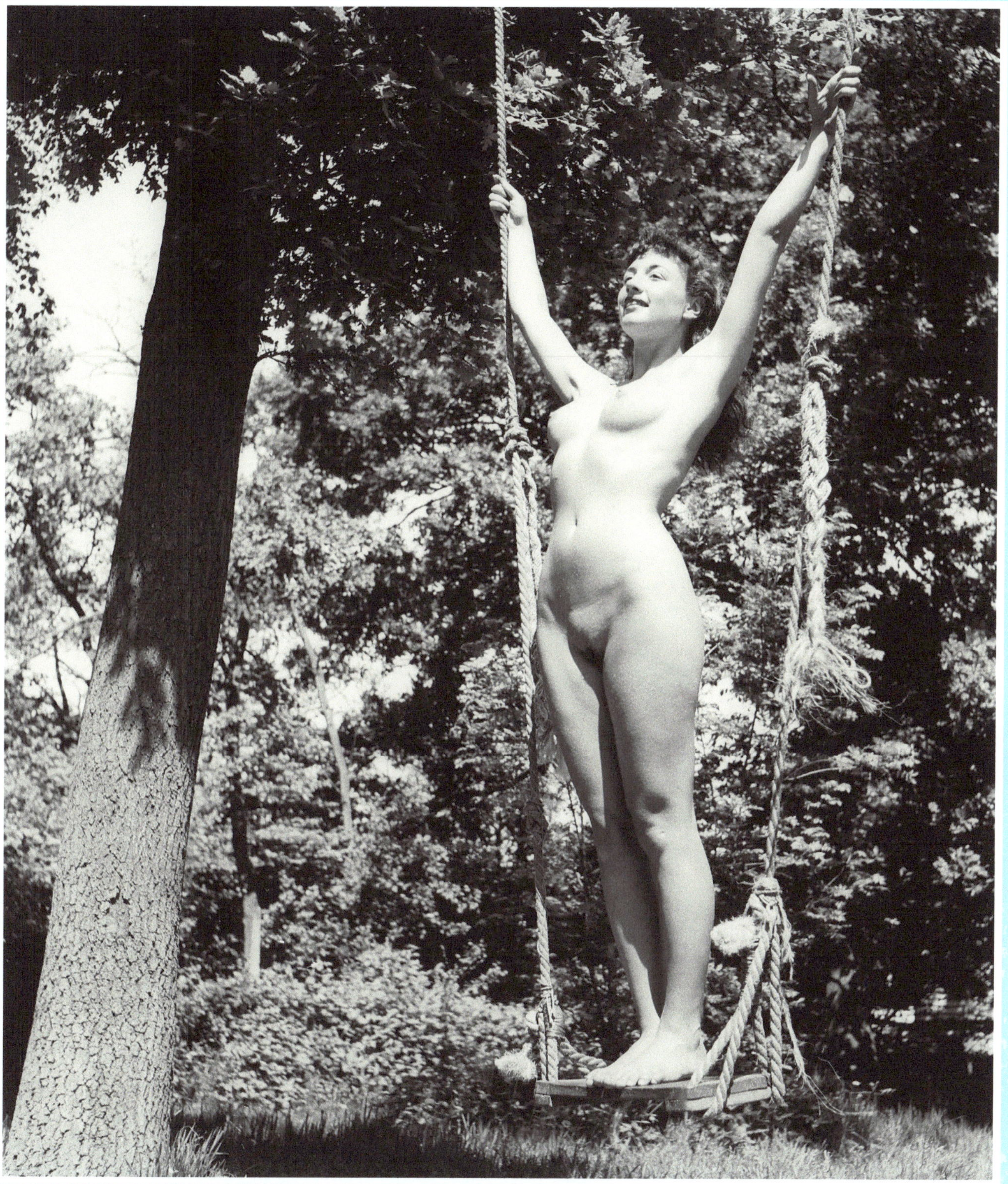

Left and above: Pamela Green, photographed in the grounds of Spielplatz. The image on the left featured in *Health and Efficiency* magazine in January 1951 with the title "Resting Dancer".

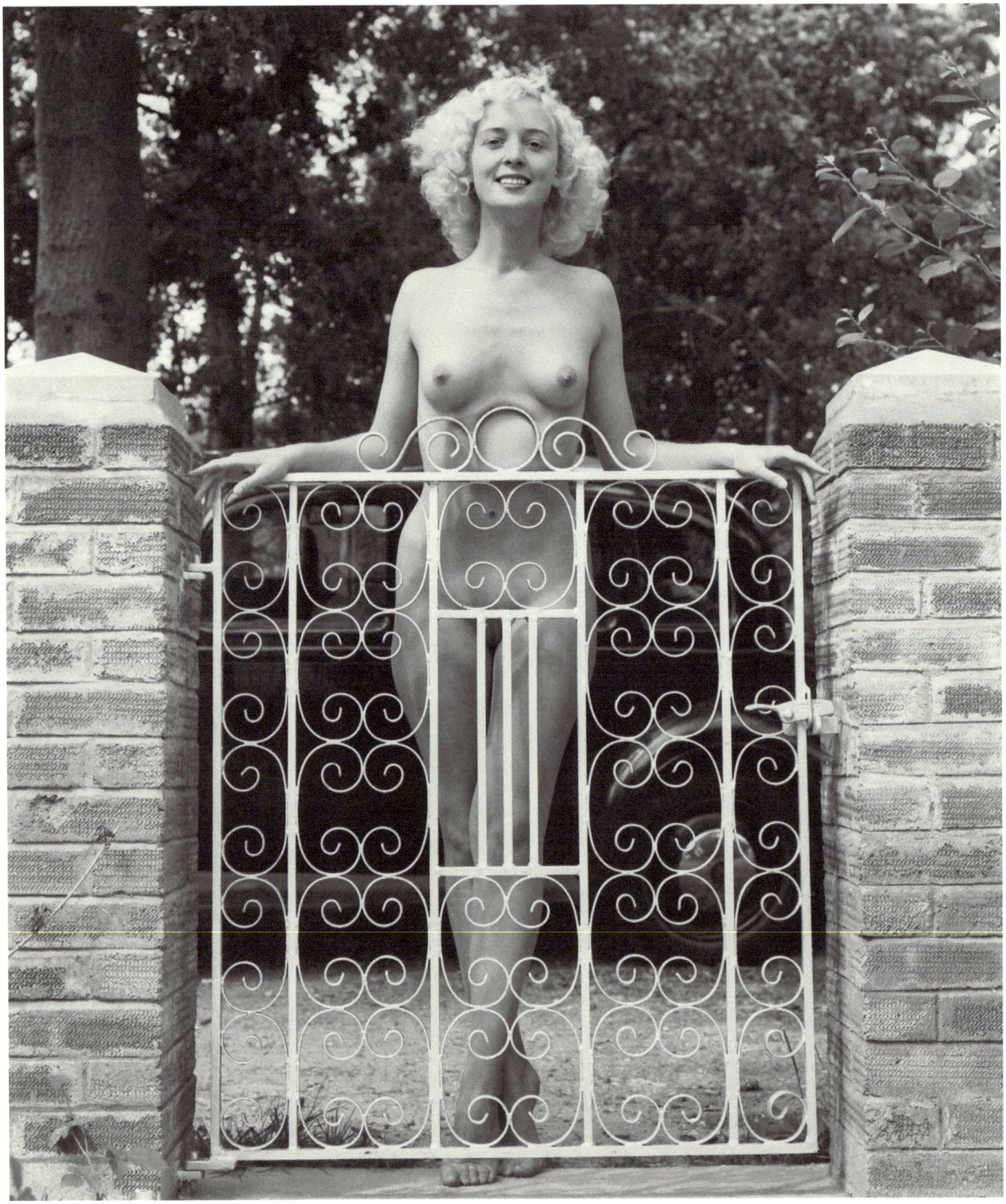

Above and right: Jean Cobb.

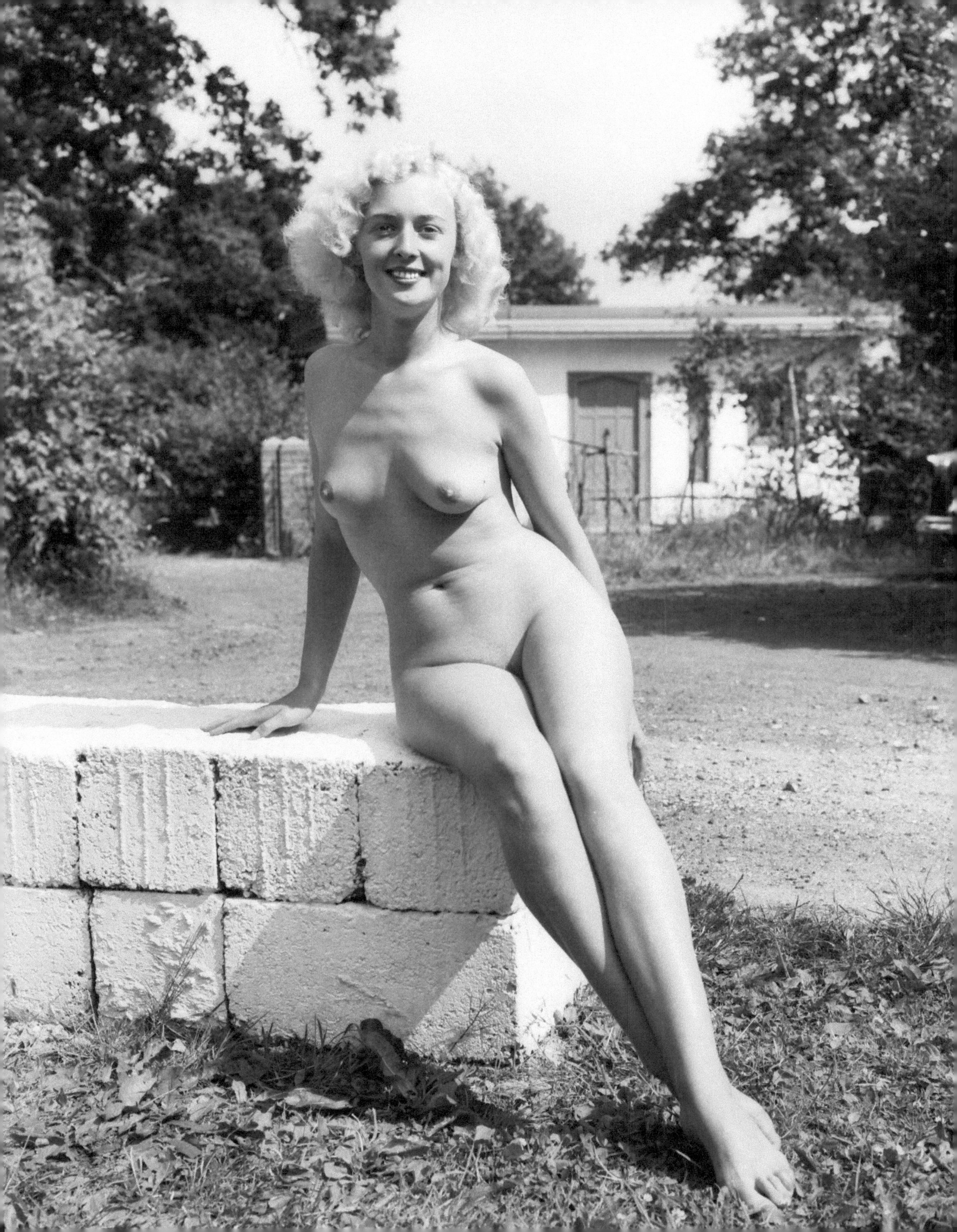

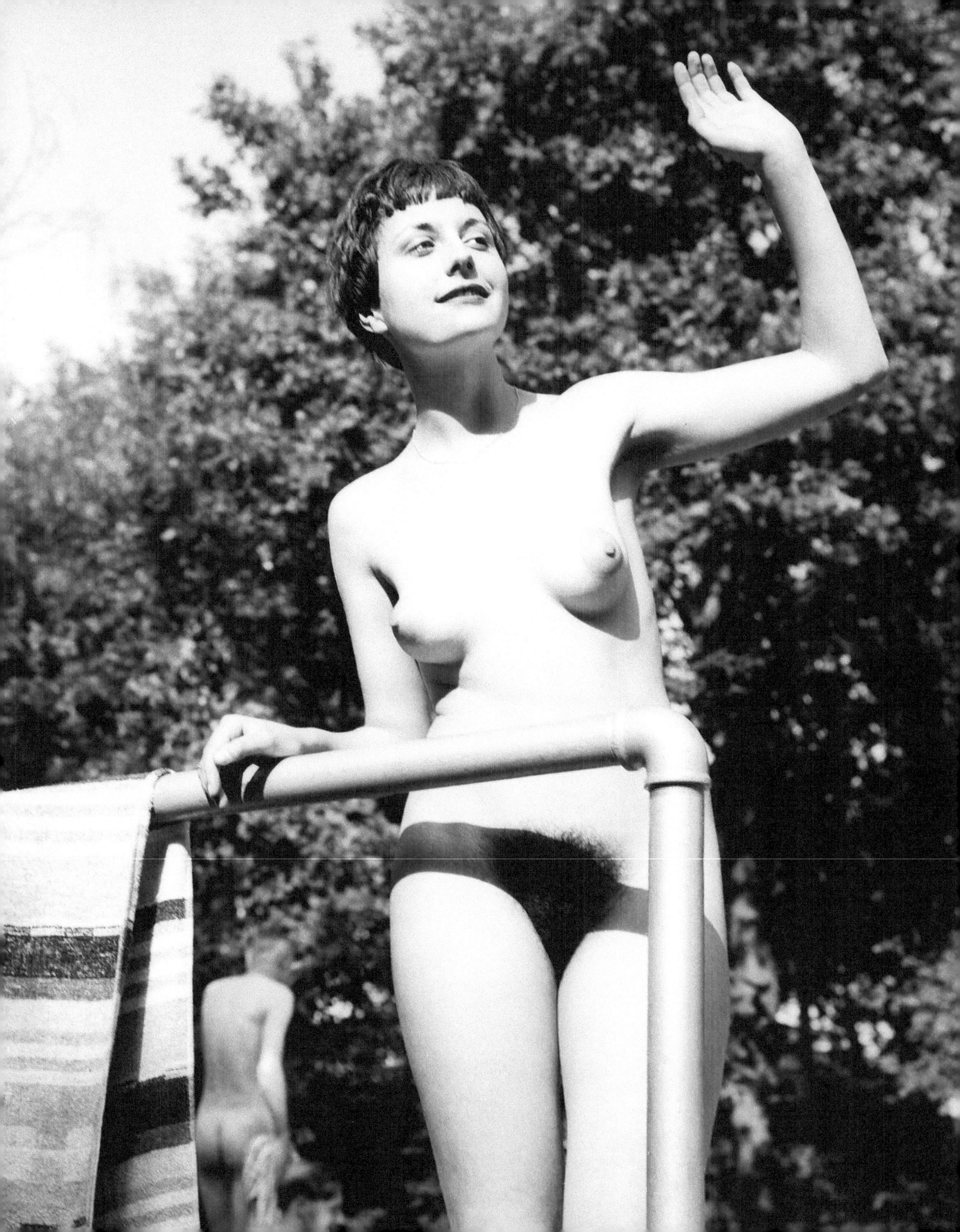

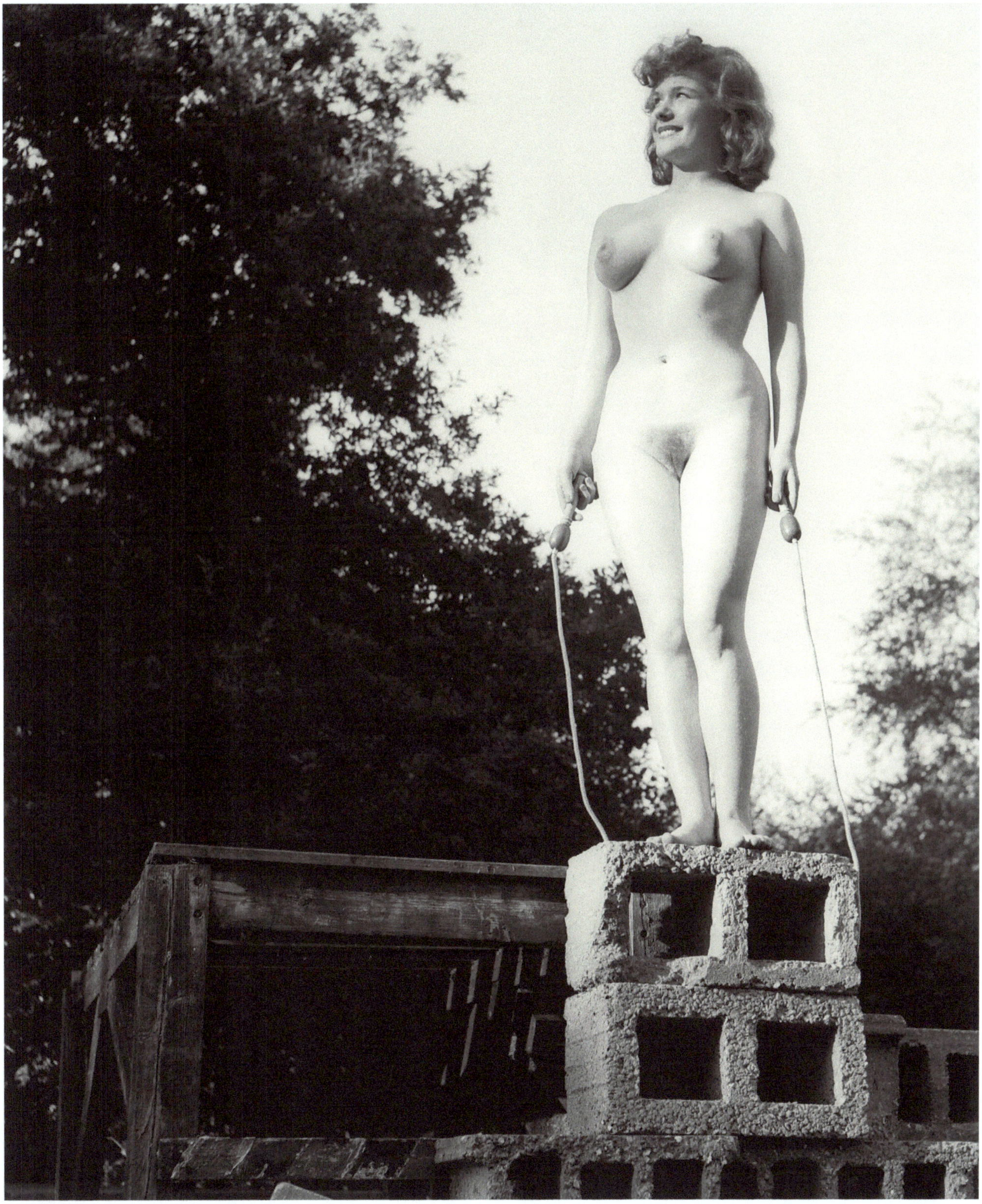

Above: The dangerous art of skipping nude while balancing on a pile of breeze blocks.

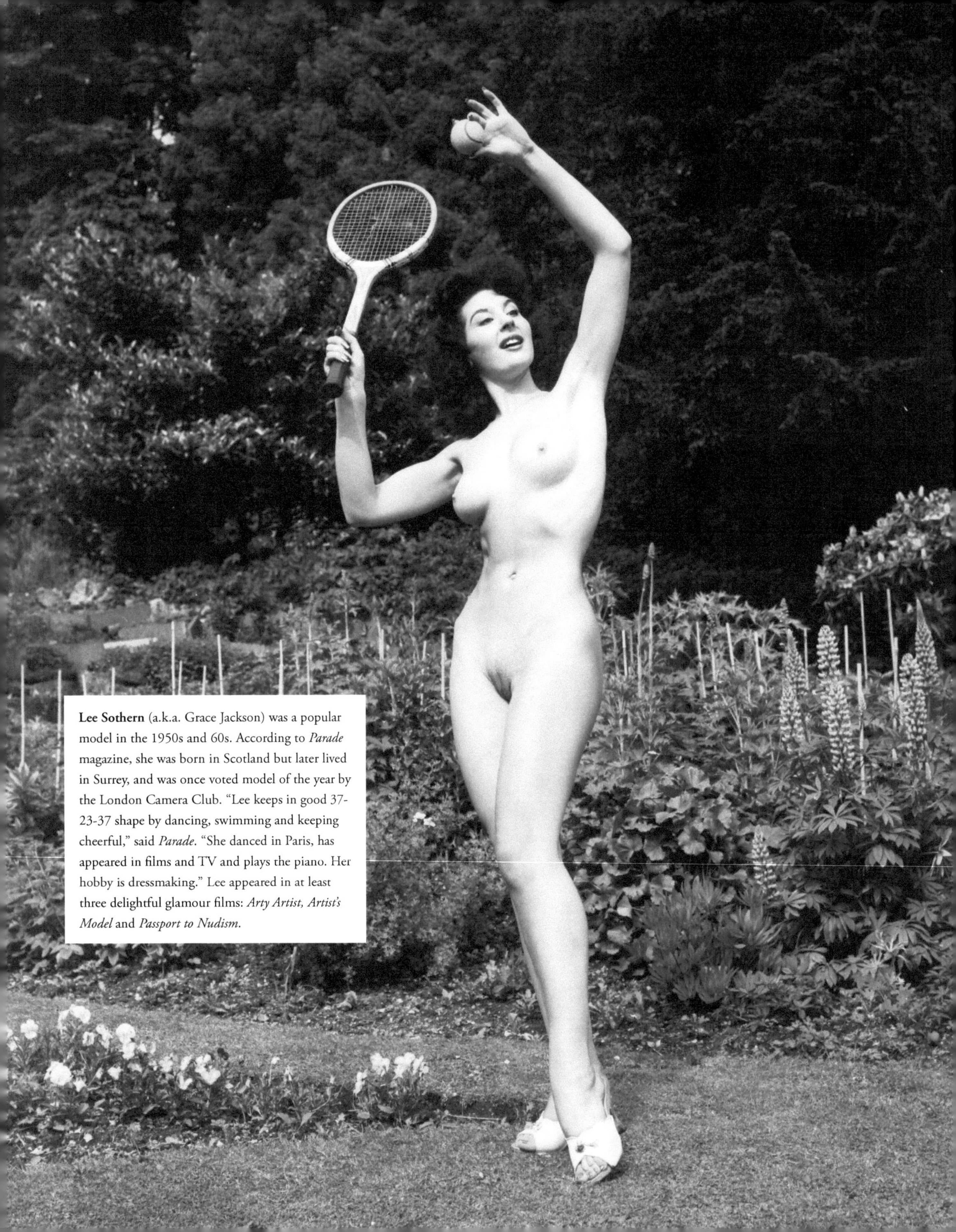

Lee Sothern (a.k.a. Grace Jackson) was a popular model in the 1950s and 60s. According to *Parade* magazine, she was born in Scotland but later lived in Surrey, and was once voted model of the year by the London Camera Club. "Lee keeps in good 37-23-37 shape by dancing, swimming and keeping cheerful," said *Parade*. "She danced in Paris, has appeared in films and TV and plays the piano. Her hobby is dressmaking." Lee appeared in at least three delightful glamour films: *Arty Artist, Artist's Model* and *Passport to Nudism*.

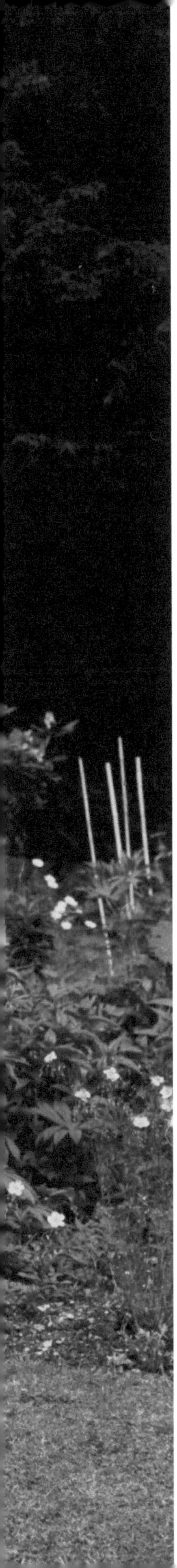

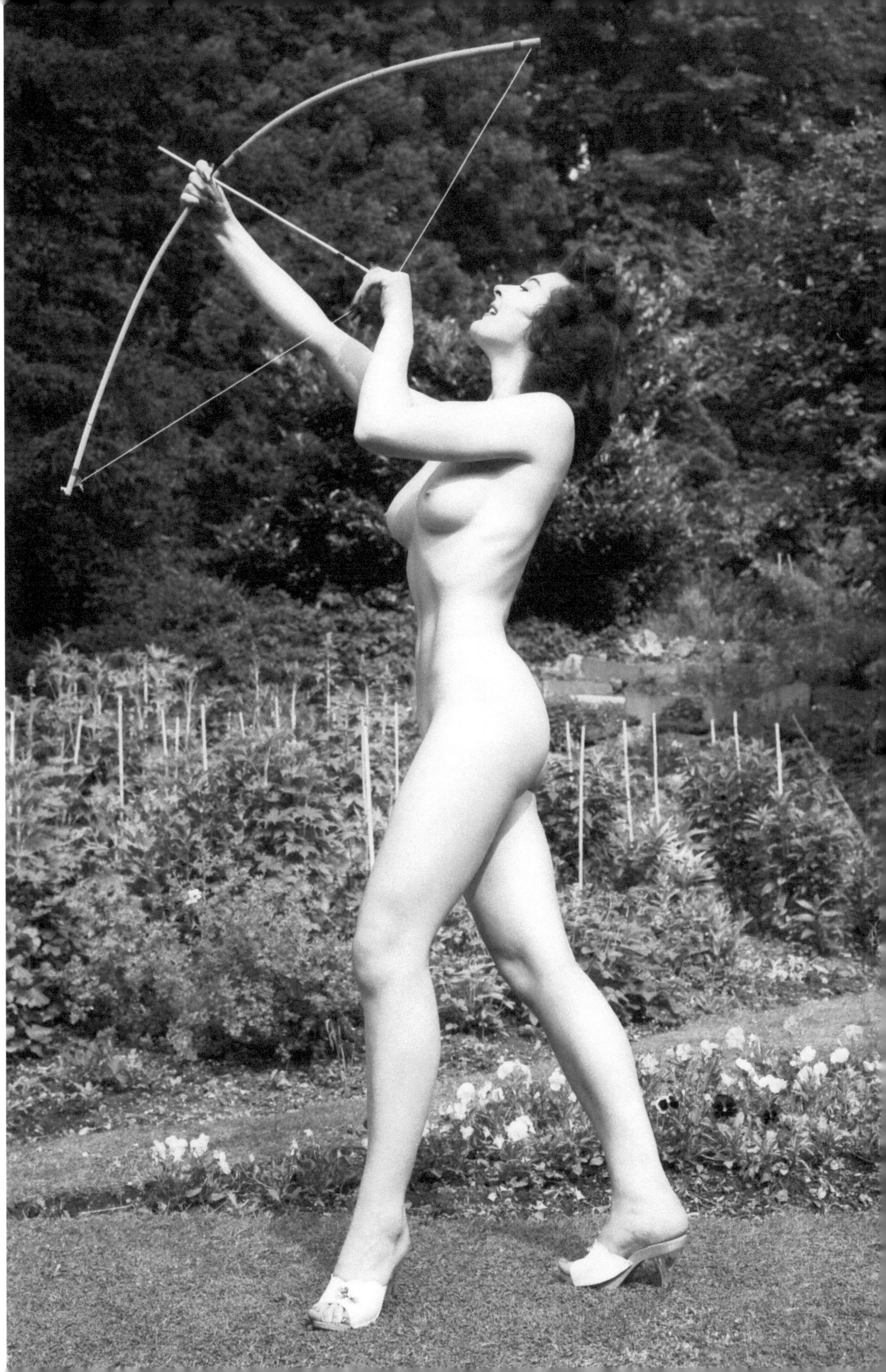

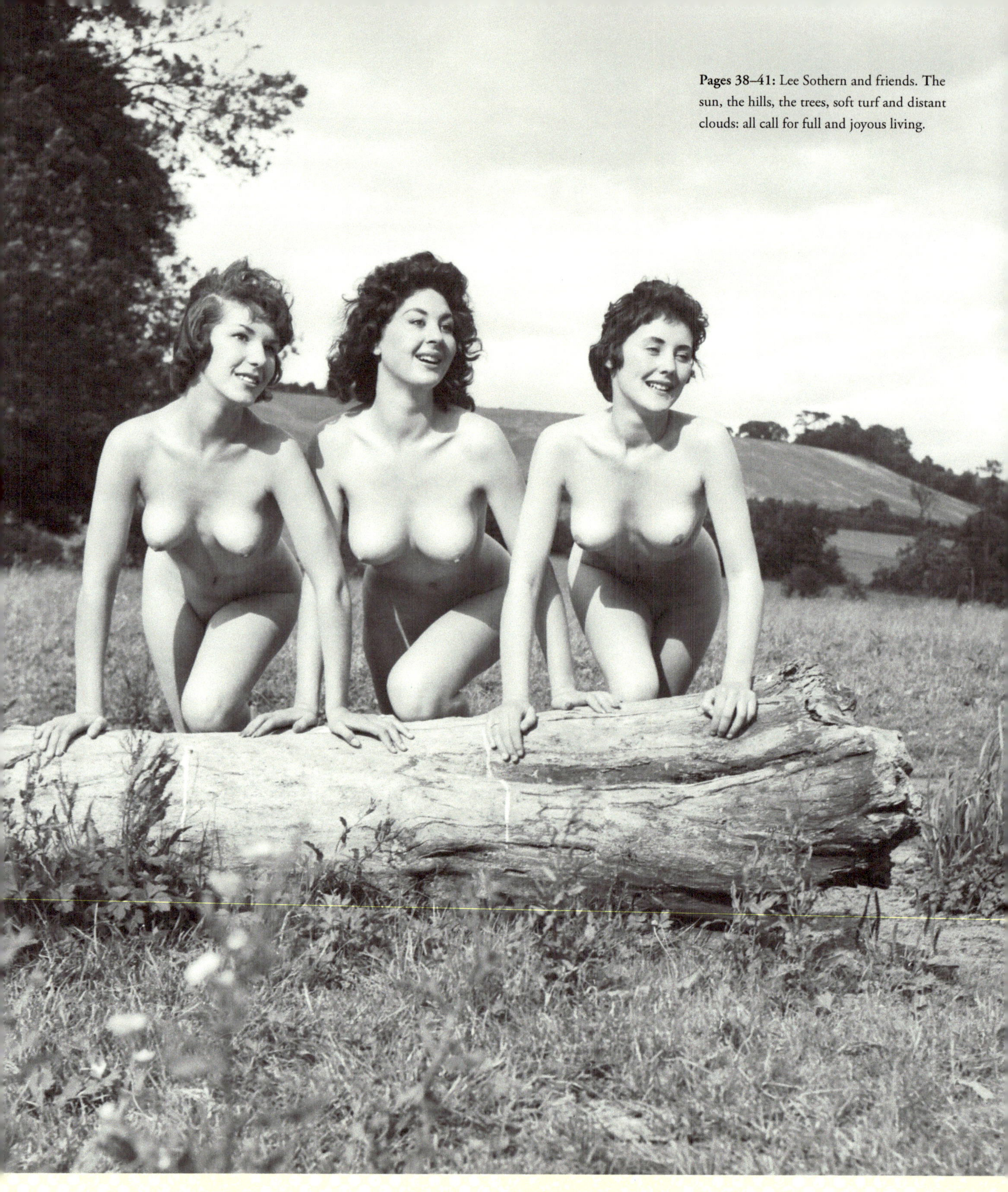

Pages 38–41: Lee Sothern and friends. The sun, the hills, the trees, soft turf and distant clouds: all call for full and joyous living.

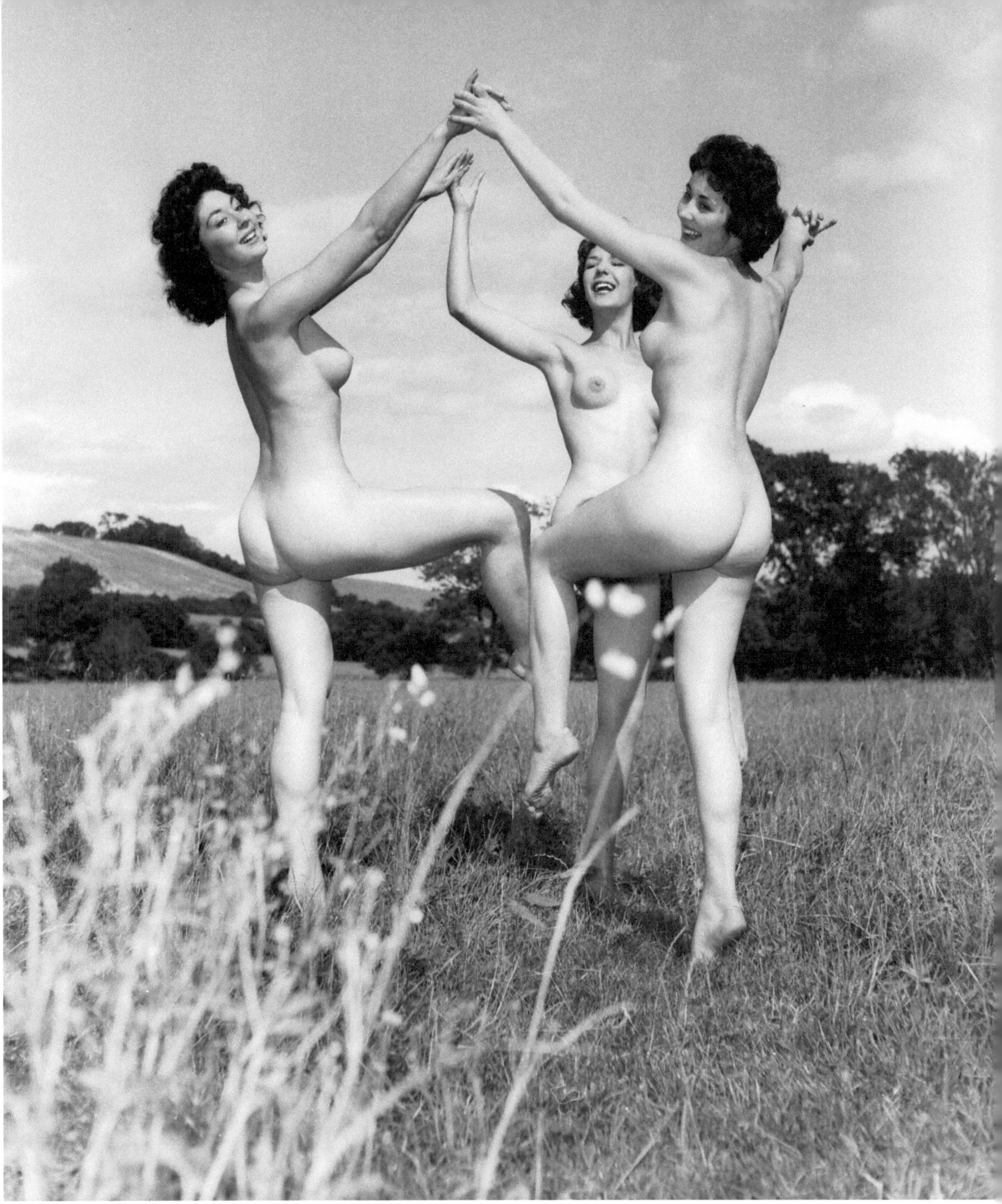

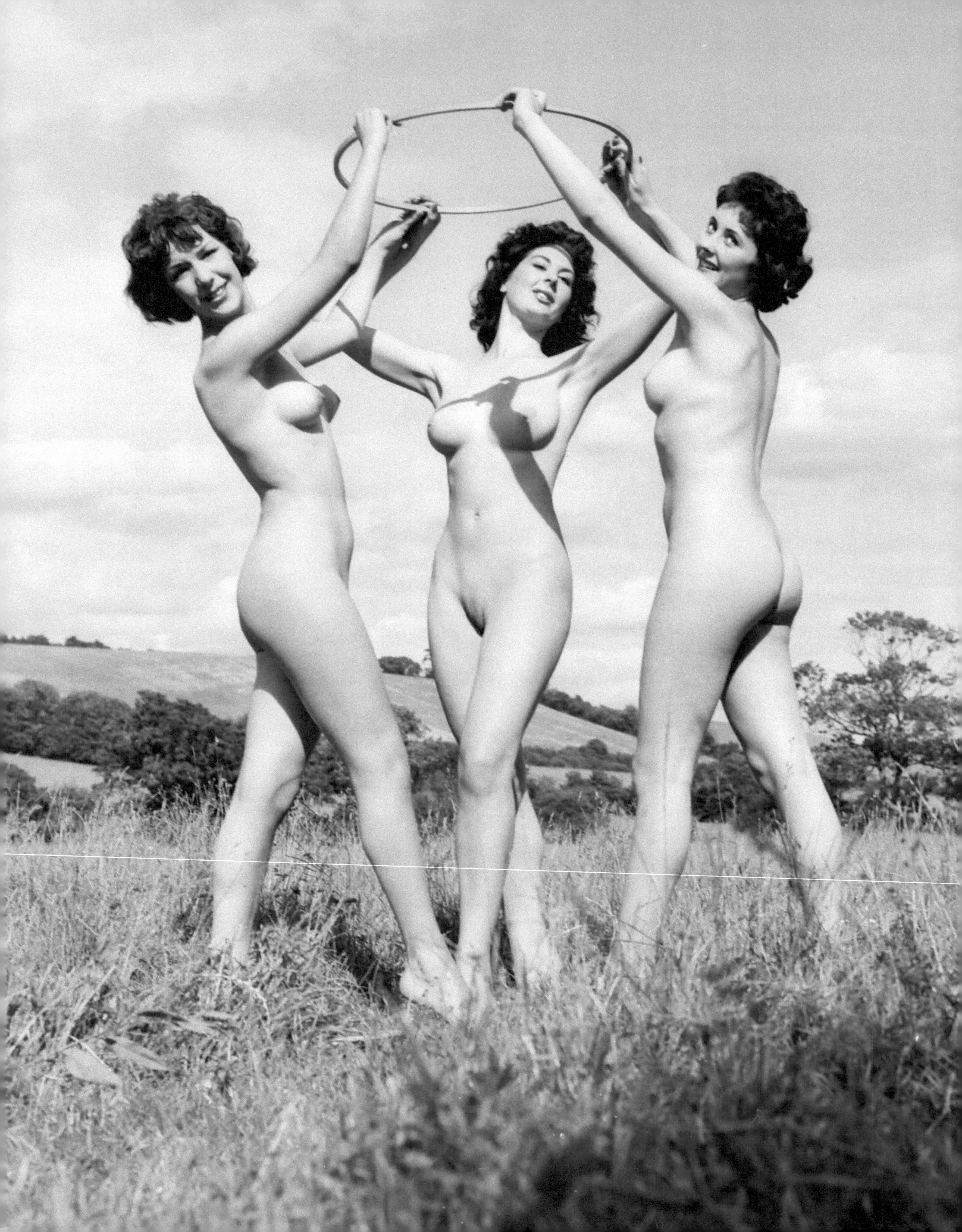

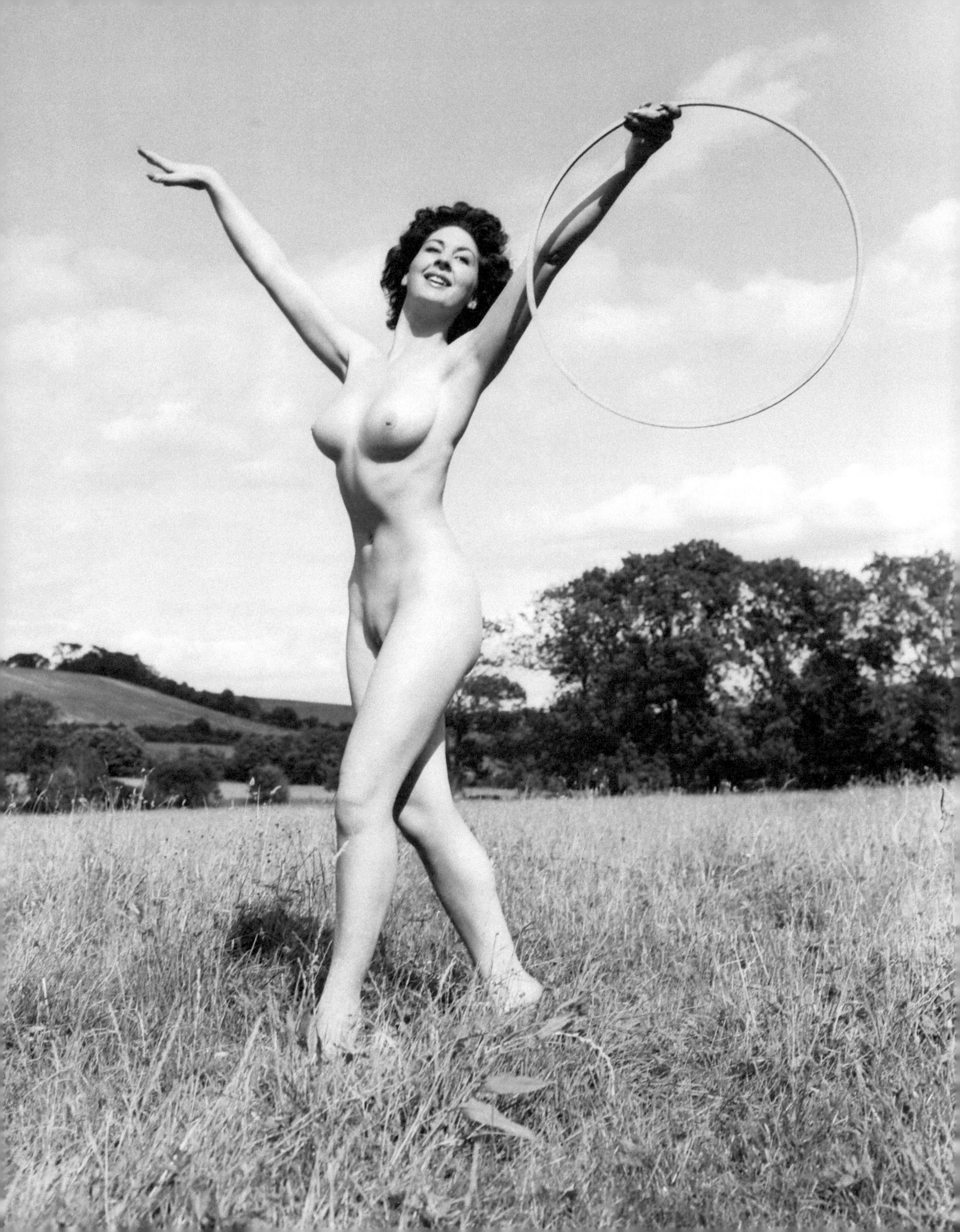

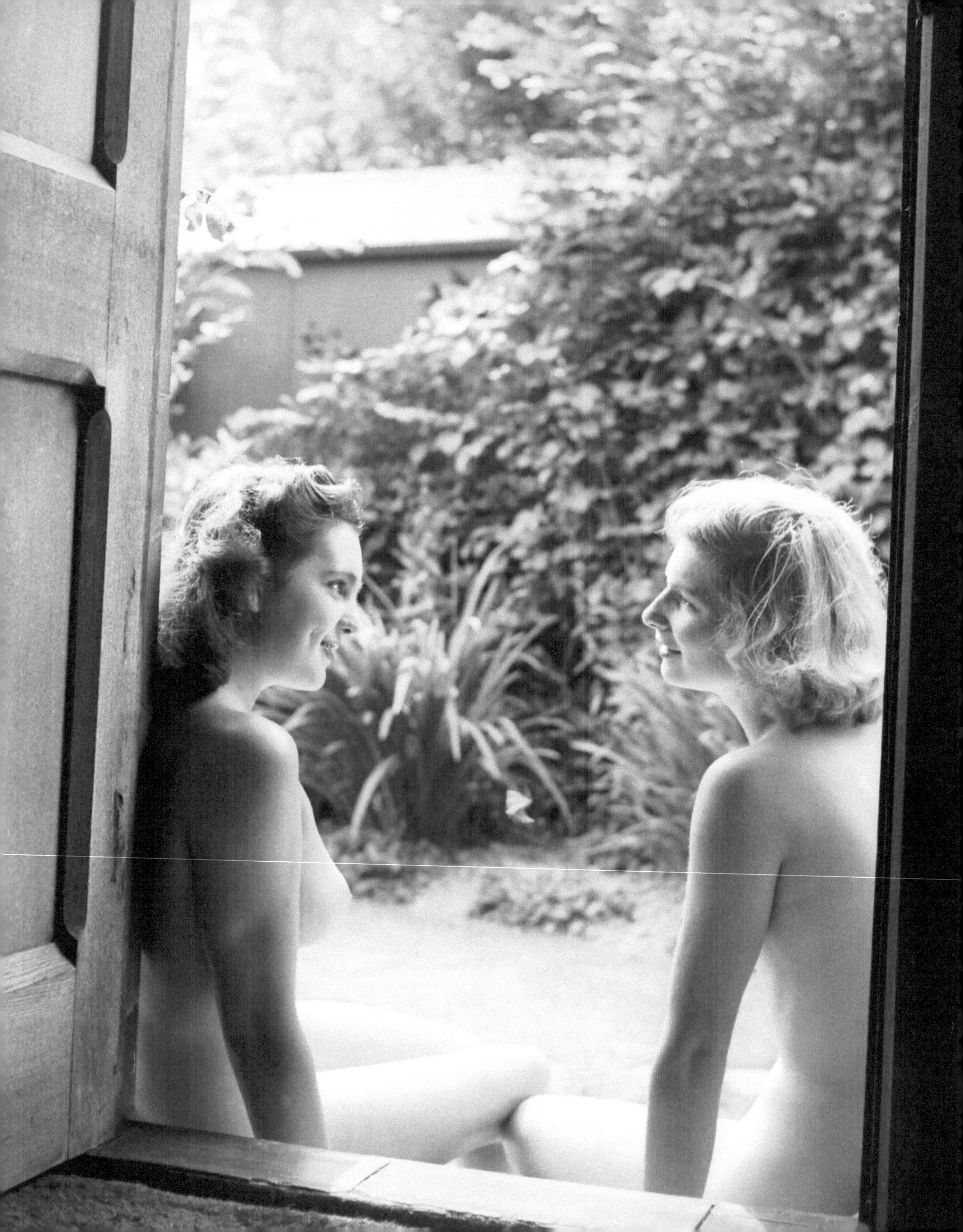

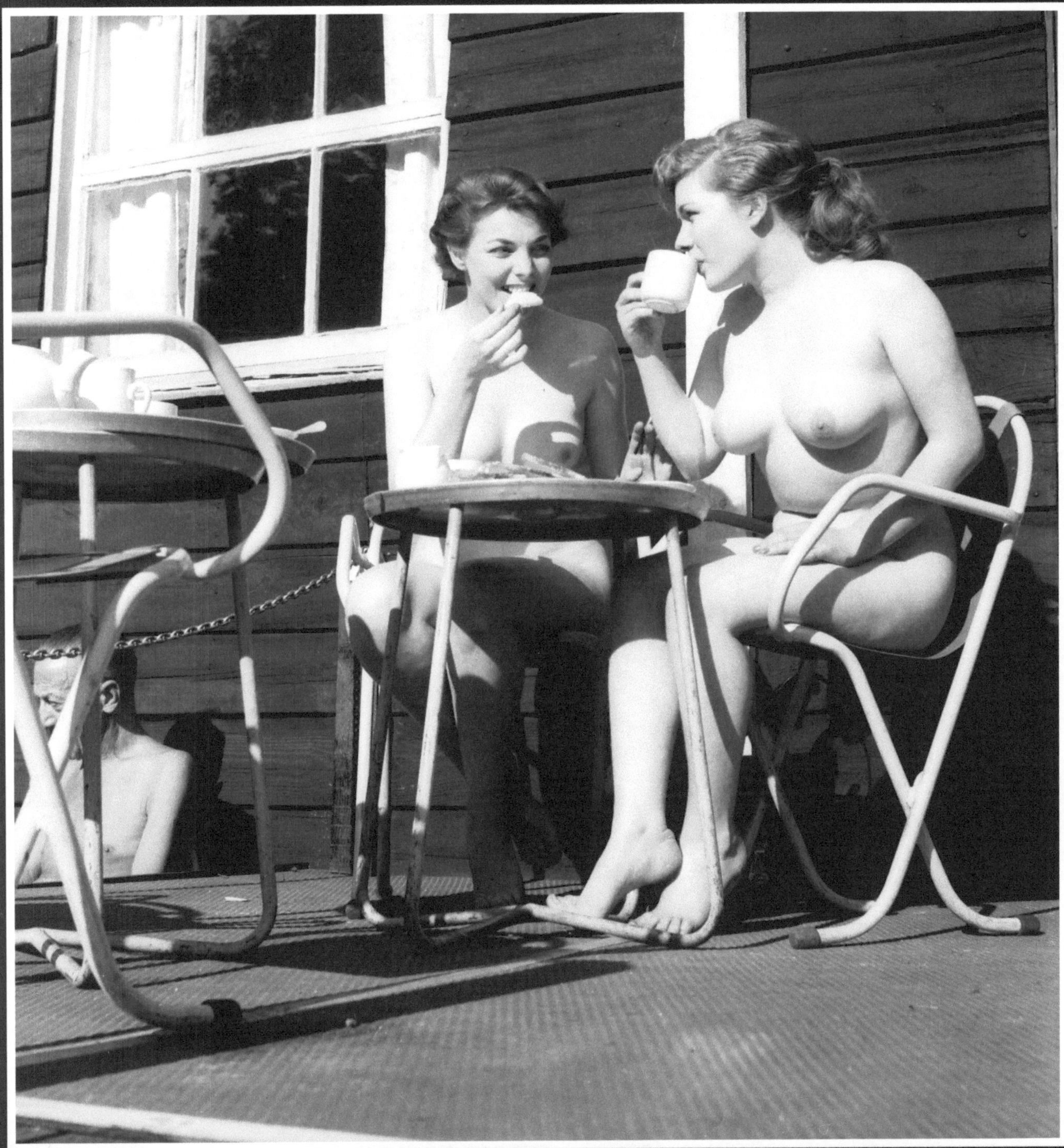

Above: Tea for two outside the club house at Spielplatz naturist village.

Left: Audrey Goodman and Beryl Sidey.

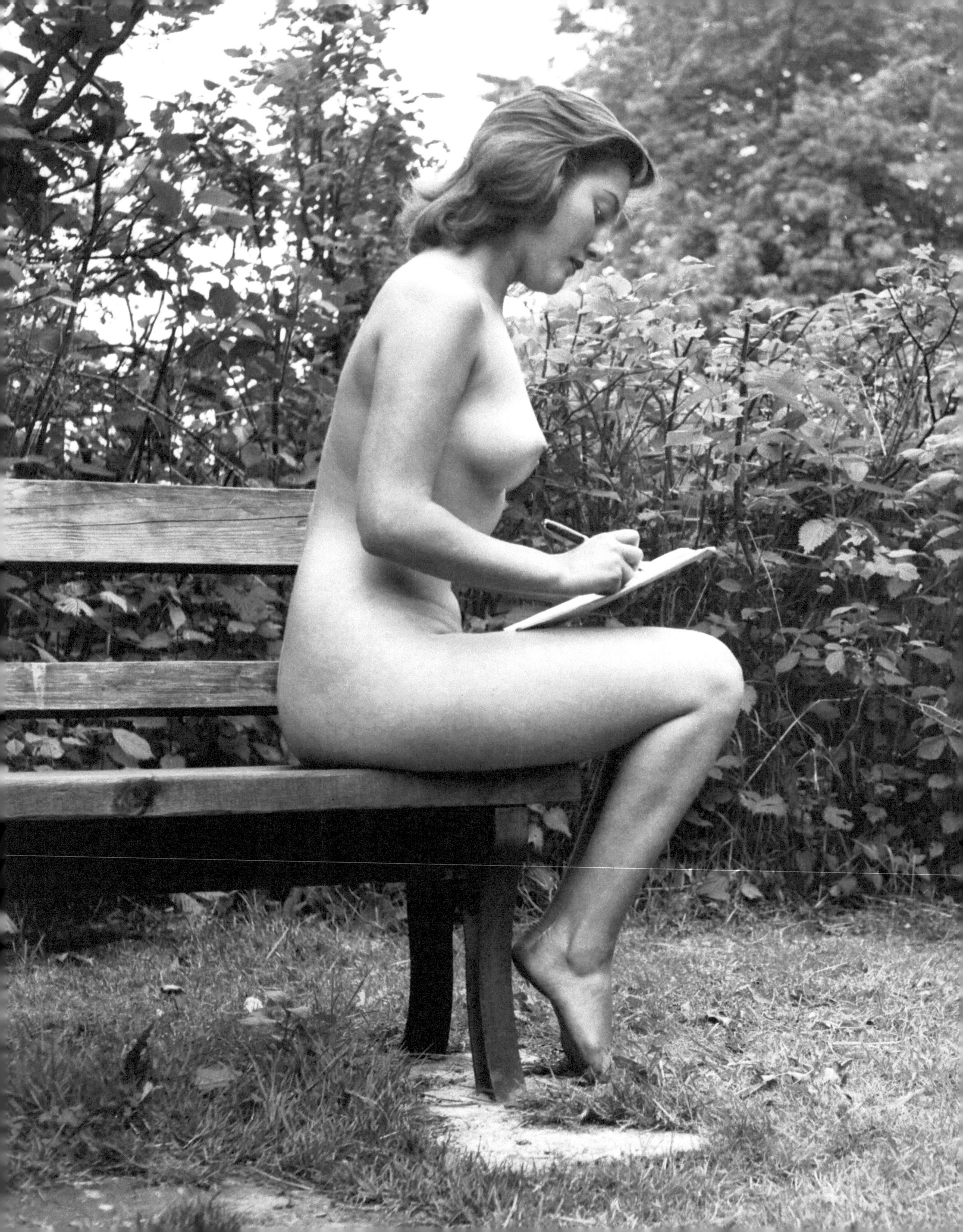

AVAILABLE TITLES FROM WOLFBAIT

Doing Rude Things
The history of the British sex film.

NEW!
Cinema au Naturel
A history of nudist film.

Miniten: Rules of the Game
Invented in the 1930s, Miniten is a tennis-like game played by naturists.

Naked as Nature Intended
The epic tale of a nudist picture by Pamela Green, with photographs by Douglas "Dambuster" Webb, DFM.

The Naked Truth About Harrison Marks
The notorious biography by Franklyn Wood.

Past Masters of the Nude
An illustrated bibliography of nude photography books published in England from 1896 to 1960.

THE STEPHEN GLASS COLLECTION

Amazons of Yesteryear
A rare, action-packed collection of images of wrestling women of the 1940s and 1950s.

Beauty Off-Duty
Relaxed, everyday moments caught on camera.

Naked in the Menagerie
A playful look at Eve accompanied by her animal friends.

Nudist Camp Follies – volumes 1 and 2
An intimate look at the natural and free atmosphere in Sun Clubs.

Nymphs and Naiads
Beauty unadorned and outdoors.

NEW!
Poise and Pose
A magnificent series of photographs of female beauty taken in the studio.

Order online at wolfbait.co.uk

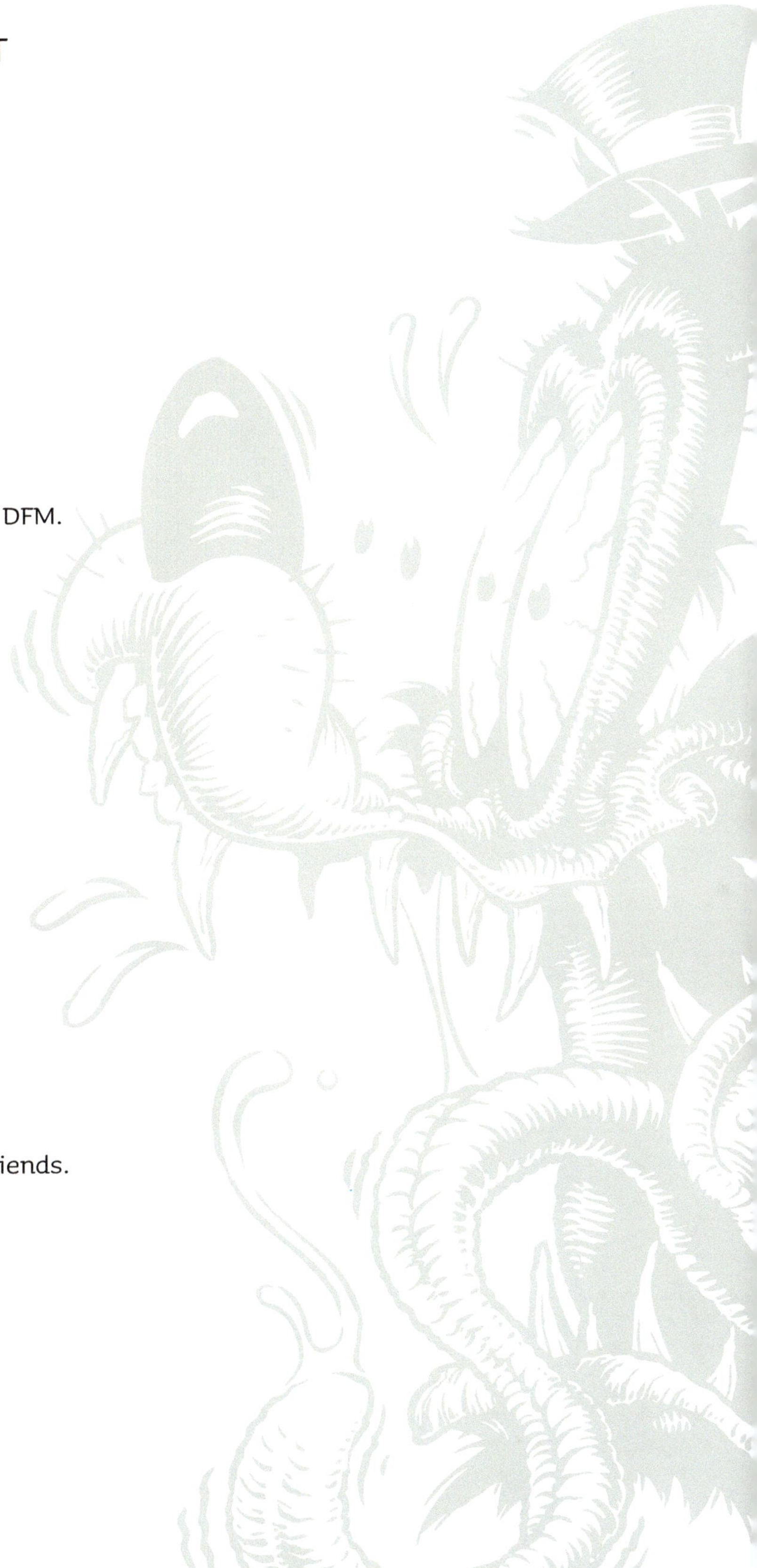

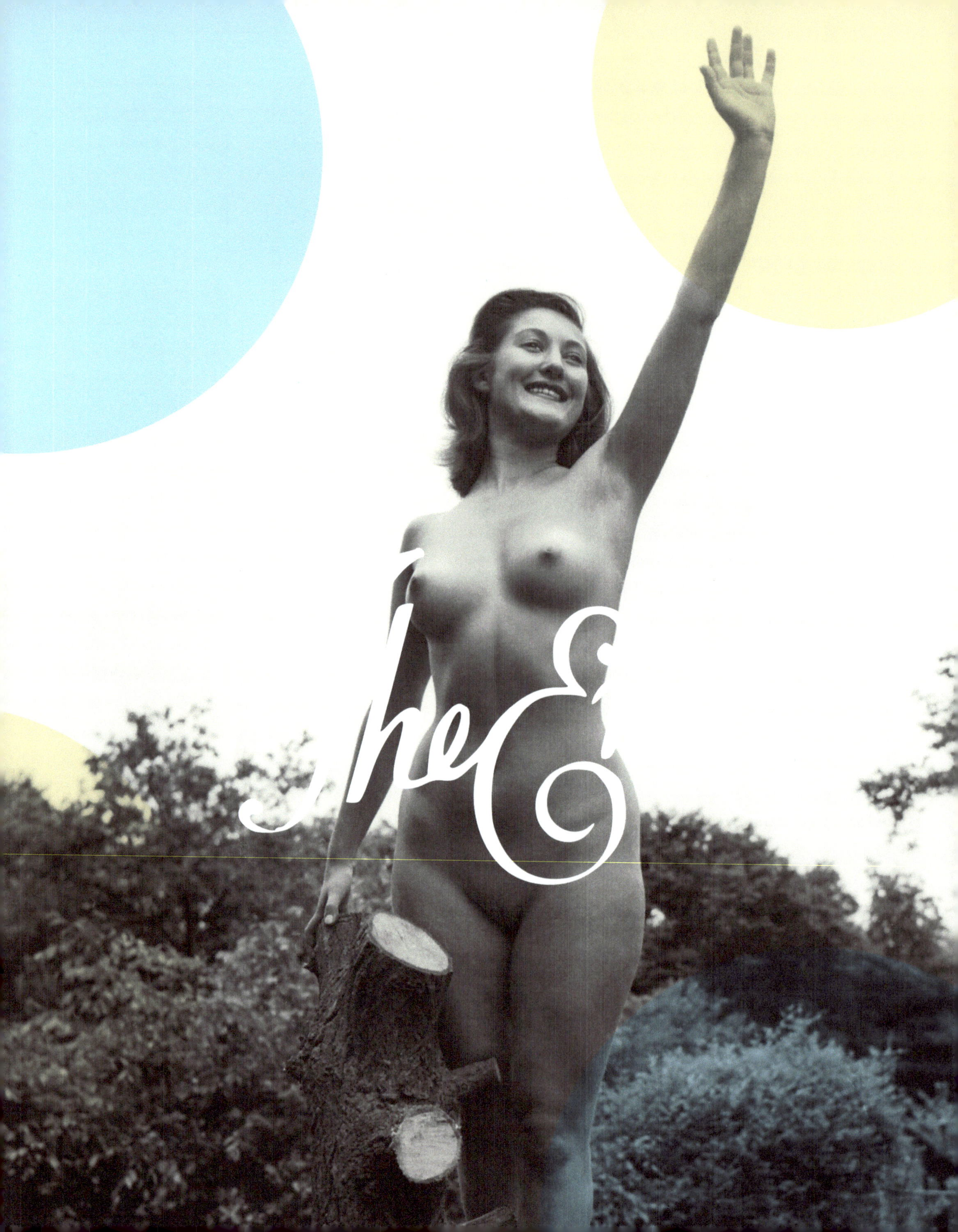